WE'RE WORKING OUT:

A Zen Approach to Everyday Fitness

By Al Kavadlo, CSCS

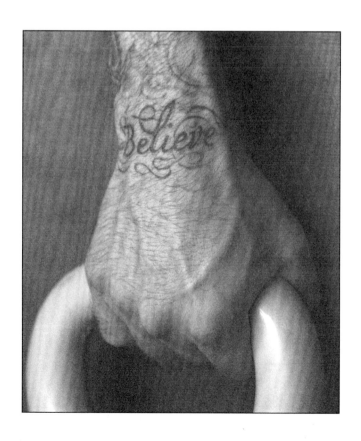

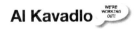

We're Working Out:
A Zen Approach to Everyday Fitness

ISBN 978-0-615-37438-3

Graphic design: Perceive Creative (www.perceivecreative.com)

Cover photo and concept: Dan Budiac

Back cover photo: Chris Shonting

Inside photos: Chris Shonting and Dan Budiac

All indoor photos taken at Nimble Fitness (www.NimbleFitness.com)

Editing: Amy Shigo and Travis Rave

For more information visit www.AlKavadlo.com

Published by Muscle-Up Books

Disclaimer

The ideas and opinions discussed in this book are intended for educational and entertainment purposes only. This book is not intended to replace medical advice, nor to diagnose or treat any condition, illness or injury. Furthermore, Al Kavadlo is not liable for any injuries or damages that individuals might incur by attempting to perform any of the exercises or feats of strength depicted or discussed in this book. Any individual attempting to does so at their own risk. Consult with a licensed physician before beginning an exercise regimen.

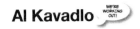

Al Kavadlo

Acknowledgments

Thank you to Carl, Rosalie, Danny and Jesse Kavadlo, Amy Shigo, Travis Rave, Chris Shonting, Shir Konas, Dan Budiac, Armen Gemdjian, Matt Dellapina, Mike Lieberman, Daniel Lucas, Keith Paine, Antonio Sini, Erica Vichnes, Emma Robinson, Karen Smyers, Kirsten Kincade, Meng He, Rick Seedman, Amanda Len, Kartik Tamhane, Liz Frankel, Barbara Fierman, Virginia Webb, Lenny Lefebrve, Ron Hamilton, Randy Humola, Larry Gruber, Calvin Vickers, Cherise Compobasso, Jeff Bodnar, Ed Helfer, Trish Balbert, Kenneth Cappello, John O'Mahoney, Elliot Rechtin, Shera Strange, Eric Bergmann, Matt Ruskin, Matt Moses, Greg Samothrakis, Julia Forte and all my other friends, colleagues and clients who have supported and believed in me over the years. This book would not have been possible without your help and support!

Table of Contents

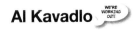

Foreward

I began my career as a personal trainer in 2003 and got my first paid gig as a fitness writer/expert in 2006. I was hired as a columnist for the companion website to *Younger Next Year*, a non-fiction bestseller at the time. I wrote a lot of articles for them over the next several months. During this time I started working on a piece (which would eventually become this book) about applying the precepts of Zen Buddhism to everyday fitness. I kept it to myself, knowing that someday I would come back to it.

In the meantime, my personal training business was starting to take off and writing wasn't paying that well. When faced with the decision to put aside writing or turn down paying clients, I chose to focus on training. Funny thing is, clients kept asking me when I was going to write a book!

Eventually the day came when I left my corporate personal training job to go totally independent. I referred many of my clients to other trainers and got down to writing. This book and my blog (www.AlKavadlo.com) have since taken up as much of my life as my personal training business.

A lot of people helped me along the way (see previous page) and countless hours went into making this book, yet I am amazed that as I give it one last look over, there are still things in here that I want to change! In the exercise section, for example, I don't mention trunk rotation as a fundamental movement and I probably should have. I stuck a couple of pictures in there to try to make up for it though. I also don't mention the importance of getting a good night's sleep, so I'm doing it now. The whole "early to bed, early to rise" thing really works. I'm sure I'll find more problems as I look back on this book each time, but that's life.

And that's pretty much the whole idea behind this book: nothing is ever finished, there is always room for growth. Keeping a fresh perspective and questioning your beliefs—especially your closest held beliefs—allows you to experience that growth. Change is not something to fear or to feel foolish about. To paraphrase a quote that's attributed to Buddha, "there are only two mistakes one can make: not starting and not going all the way."

Since you've read this far, you've already started! Are you ready to go all the way?

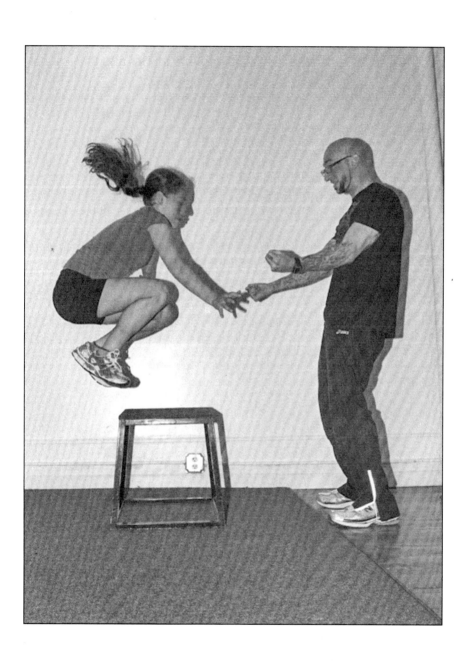

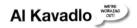
Al Kavadlo

A No-Nonsense Introduction

I was a tall, scrawny kid growing up in Brooklyn and I didn't want to get my ass kicked, so once I was thirteen I decided to start lifting weights. I still remember my mom taking me to a store called Consumers to get my first set of weights and seeing the man wheel the box out from the stock room on a hand truck. The set was so heavy that we needed him to help us get everything in the car! I got more serious about lifting throughout high school and opting to take weight training as my phys. ed. credit was a great way to get out of playing actual sports (like I said, I was lanky and unathletic).

When I was eighteen I was desperate to bulk up and a crafty salesman at GNC took advantage of that emotion. I purchased a product called Testrogel, an exercise supplement that claimed to increase testosterone production when rubbed onto your skin prior to exercise. This (supposed) testosterone boost would not only give you extra strength during your workout, but also claimed to help with muscle growth and the recovery process. Finally there was something that could make me big and strong! My days of being puny were over, at least in theory. The reality of the product was that it did absolutely nothing, except teach me a valuable lesson about gullibility.

In college I got interested in bodybuilding. At that time, I was still just concerned with aesthetics. I wanted to get diesel! This led me to do research about how the body works. As I got more and more into fitness, a career in personal training seemed like the obvious choice. It was also around this time that I first discovered Zen Buddhism. Over the years, my interest in Eastern philosophy has greatly impacted the way that I approach fitness. Instead of living in a fantasy world of musclemen with flawless physiques and perfect smiles, my focus was now grounded in reality. I wasn't a hulking bodybuilder but that didn't stop me from becoming a successful trainer. I've trained many people, including athletes, models, the elite business class and even an Olympic medalist.

I'm not going to bullshit you: getting fit isn't easy. We live in a society that relies on consumption and encourages abundance. People drive their cars to the end of the driveway to pick up their mail. We super-size our meal and then eat it in front of the TV. In short, we live in the FATTEST country in the world. Yet in spite of all this, millions of Americans are in fantastic shape. That's right, millions of Americans are fit! Surprising, right? But it's true—lots of us are lean and mean, and you can be, too. Seriously. That's why you're reading this, isn't it?

Every year millions of people begin a new exercise plan in an attempt to lose weight and most of them fail. They reach for the next new thing and hope that this time will be different. People are constantly seeking out the newest fad diets and exercise programs in hopes that they will find some miracle weight loss solution or the holy grail of workout regimens. Why is it then that the majority of Americans remain overweight and out of shape? It comes down to the fact that most people cannot stick to an exercise regimen and healthy diet for the long term. They look for shortcuts and make excuses, hoping someday things will be different, easier. They wait (sitting on their couches and eating their pie) for the miracle cure, the magical program that requires no effort and guarantees results. But the fact of the matter is, that program doesn't exist and it probably never will. However, there is a tried and true method out there that people have been using for quite some time and I guarantee you, it works. Of course, I'm talking about the combination of a healthy diet and a serious, consistent exercise program.

One of the major problems with getting fit is that it's so easy to find someone that's worse off than you. All you have to do is go to the grocery store and look around. On your right, there's someone filling up his cart with soda and potato chips. On the left, there's a lady turning sideways in order to squeeze by your cart. In such an environment, it's easy to think, "Wow, that person is even fatter than I am." It's common to think, "I could be so much worse. At least I'm not THAT big." When there are constantly people around who are in worse shape than you, it's easy to use them as an excuse, but that's not the best way to feel better about yourself. What you need to remember is that there is another side of the spectrum. Sure there are people who are bigger than you, but there are also loads of people who are fitter and healthier than you. The first thing you need to do is change your mindset. Concentrate on yourself instead of looking at those who are less fit. If you need to compare yourself to someone else then look to those who are doing it, those who are fitter and healthier, those who have implemented a healthy diet and exercise regimen and made a positive transformation. Look at them and ask yourself this, "Are they better than me?"

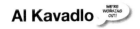

Before answering that, just think about it for a second. Are they really capable of something that you are not? Are they really better than you?

Now, as you look at some toned, young woman or some ripped guy, various negative thoughts will probably start running through your head—reasons why you don't believe in yourself, how you're at some disadvantage. You'll make up excuses—genetics maybe, or some old injury. Or maybe just plain, old laziness. And then you'll whine, "You don't understand!" But I do understand; I'm not any better than anyone else. Not the fit guy or the slim woman, not the potato chip guy or the squeezing lady and certainly not you. I never had it any easier than any of you and neither did anybody else.

So while such negative thoughts are natural, you don't have to give into them! I won't grant you any excuses because there are countless, ordinary people who've overcome adversity and gone on to accomplish unbelievable things. It's not easy, but it's worth it.

Not what you wanted to hear? Tough. I told you I wasn't going to bullshit you. The first challenge is to rebel against the part of your psyche that doesn't think you can do it. The reason many people can't stick with a program for the long term is because of the people themselves. We're often our own worst enemy. Everyone reading this book already knows what to do; you're probably just having a hard time following through with it. People think to themselves, "That diet didn't work" or "This exercise program isn't working," but really it's the people that aren't working. If you really want to get fit and be healthy, you need to accept that it is totally up to you. You have to do it. No one else can do it for you. Others can help—we can motivate you, support you and try our best to keep you in check—but at the end of the day, it is you and only you that can really do anything about it.

Now don't start getting defensive over there. The idea that you (and only you) are responsible for your own circumstances is not something to fear. It is actually an incredibly empowering concept once you put it into practice. If this sounds harsh, remember that you're at a place now where every fit person has been: the beginning. This doesn't necessarily mean that you've never been to the gym or never run any farther than the mailbox. If you haven't, that's fine—this book will help you. If personal fitness is something you've been working on but you just need help focusing—this book will help you. If you're already an experienced and fit person, but you're looking for a different approach or a more effective regimen—this book will help you. It's important to remember that in some respects, we are all beginners. Do your best to stay humble and focused. You can do this. You will do this. This book will help you to find your inner strength and then show you how to put that strength into action. I will guide you away from the distracting elements in your life and bring you deeper into yourself. I will show you how to actually enjoy exercise and fitness. For without joy, you stand little chance at continued success. Most of all, I will show you, YOU, and you may be surprised by what you see.

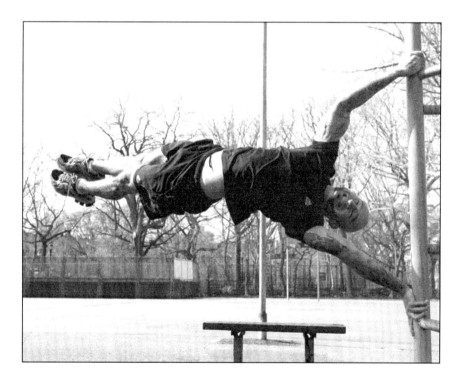

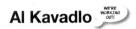
Chapter One:
The First is the Worst

When it comes to exercising, people are filled with excuses. I've heard everything from "I'm just not athletic" to "I'm big boned, so what's the point?" I've even heard people whine, "Well then I'd have to shower again." I mean, come on! What are we in 2nd grade trying to get out of doing our homework? It's ridiculous! Of course there are reasons why you won't feel like exercising, but that doesn't mean that you shouldn't. Try to recognize these rationalizations for what they are: EXCUSES.

Over the years I've learned that the hardest part of getting fit, or anything really, is getting started. When people begin a program, whether it's their first or their fiftieth, they are nervous and uncertain and often turn to the blame game. They blame work, they blame money; hell, they even blame their dogs! However, the excuse I hear most often is time. Nobody ever seems to have enough time. Now, I know you're probably a very busy person and you have a lot on your plate. There's work, bills, family obligations and loads more. But guess what? Everyone has the same problems and some of us still manage to squeeze in some exercise. How do we do it? Simple. We make it a priority. EVERYBODY HAS TIME. You just need to know where to find it. If you have time to read a book (even this one!), watch TV, surf the internet or go see a movie, then you have time to exercise. Now I'm not saying that you need to give these all up, but if you can take some of the time you've set aside for these activities and dedicate it to a workout, then you've solved your problem. My day isn't any longer than yours—twenty-four hours can go by quickly, but it doesn't take more than 15 or 20 minutes a day to start. Ask yourself this question:

Do you really believe that you can't find 15 minutes during the day
or are you just looking for a way out of doing it?

One thing I have noticed about people, and I am certainly not above this, is that
we have trouble seeing things for what they really are. We want everything to be
perfect. But if we're being honest with ourselves, we know it never will be that
easy. People chase the perfect diet and the perfect training program, believing
those things are out there somewhere, thinking that if they hold out long enough,
they'll find them. Well, I'm sorry to break it to you, but there is no perfect training
program. It isn't in this book or any other, so if that is what you are looking for, then
you're going to be continually disappointed. However, as soon as you can accept
that fitness and life are not perfect, then you'll be able to deal with them a whole
lot better. I cannot tell you how many times I've heard people put off beginning or
restarting a training program because they are waiting for everything else in life to
fall neatly into place. Unfortunately, it doesn't work like that. Life is a mess and the
chaos of our day-to-day lives will always be present in the background. Instead of
waiting for this magical, chaos-free day, we must instead embrace the chaos and
work with and around it if we are to succeed.

What does all this mean? It's simple: DON'T WAIT. There's no better day to start
than today. If you're reading this book, then fitness is on your mind. Don't fight the
urge, don't allow your brain to rationalize your laziness and don't look for excuses.
If you feel like you don't have time, then start small with 15 to 20 minute workouts
and add more in as you find more time. All in all, just do it. Today.

I know this can be an extremely tough thing to do, but take comfort in the fact that
you're not the only one. Everyone feels this way when they're starting. When new
clients of mine have trouble getting through our first workout session, I tell them:
Don't worry about it—the first is the worst. I'll remind them of that throughout the
workout. The first is the worst. I like when things rhyme.

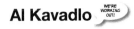

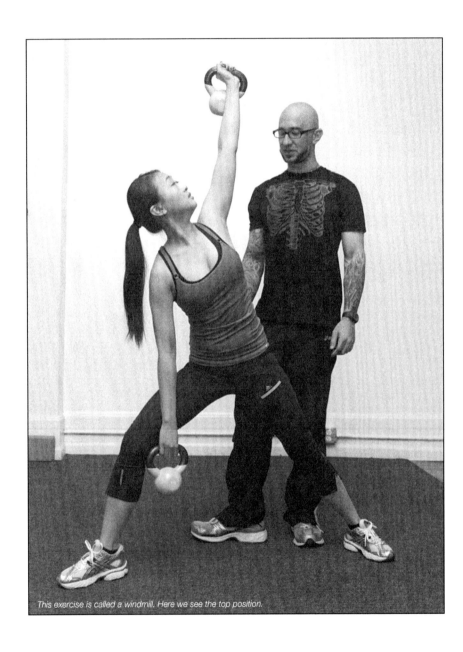

This exercise is called a windmill. Here we see the top position.

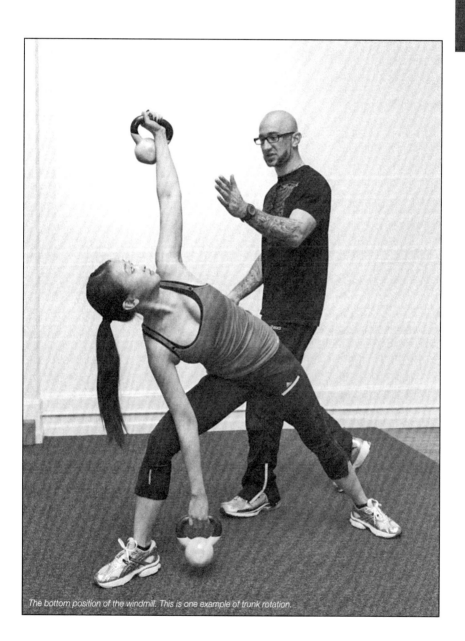

The bottom position of the windmill. This is one example of trunk rotation.

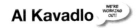

Al Kavadlo

THE DIET ISSUE

Okay, now you're mentally ready to begin, but you're not sure where to start. As I said earlier, the key to getting and staying fit is the combination of a healthy diet and a serious, consistent exercise program. I've talked briefly about how to get started exercising, but I need to discuss food as well. There are many, many diets out there and some of them are better for you than others. If you have the time and resources, you could meet with a nutritionist who would council you on changing your eating habits. But if you don't have the money or the inclination, don't worry. Here are some simple tips that, if implemented, will undoubtedly improve your diet and help you to make progress.

1. **Cut out fast food!** Let's be honest, you knew this was coming. As much as we all love to bite into a juicy double cheeseburger and then slurp it down with a cold soda, it's clearly not good for us. We all know this by now, so I'm not going to sit here and count calories for you.

   Tip: I find that I'm most tempted by fast food when I'm in a hurry. No surprise there. So next time you're pressed for time and need to grab a meal, be a little smarter with your choices. Instead of going to McDonald's or Subway (that's right—Subway is not health food!), grab a piece of fruit or a bag of mixed nuts. They're just as fast and they're significantly healthier.

2. **Eat your vegetables.** This shouldn't come as a surprise either. Our parents have been telling us this for years and they're not wrong. You should be getting at least 3-5 servings of fruits and vegetables per day—ideally more. Believe me, I know it's not as easy as it sounds. Having one good meal in the morning doesn't get you off the hook for the rest of the day (not to mention the night!). For me, daily exercise is much easier to stay on top of than healthy eating habits. I mean, if I work out in the morning, then it's done. Whatever else comes up that day, I know that I've got that workout part taken care of already. Diet is 24/7. You might give in to the occasional indulgence, but you must always be mindful of your eating habits throughout the day. I'm always surprised when I encounter people who are healthy eaters but who don't exercise consistently.

Tip: 3-5 servings might seem like a lot, I know. This is an area I personally have trouble with, too. I don't expect you to make such a huge change right away, make it gradual. Try to do more than you're doing now. If you're eating zero servings per day, try eating 1. If you're already eating 1, shoot for 2. In general, try to think in the present, in the moment. If you're out to dinner, instead of getting a side of fries, fight that urge and say no in the moment. Ask if you can substitute a salad or cooked vegetables, even if it means promising yourself that you'll get a heaping plate of fries tomorrow. Every such instance is a victory. Deal with today now and tomorrow when it comes.

3. **Limit going out to eat.** We all love going out to dinner—it's delicious and fun. Unfortunately, it's usually a little unhealthy. The portions are almost always too big and the emphasis is usually on rich taste, not nutrition.

   Tip: Don't fret, I'm not telling you to give up restaurants altogether, just try to limit it. Go out once a week instead of two or three times per week. On the other six days of the week, cook for yourself. What you make in your kitchen will almost always be healthier for you than what you would get at a restaurant and you'll also save some money (that you can put towards a trainer, gym membership or fitness gear for your home). If you hate cooking, order healthier meals from healthier places and don't feel the need to scarf it all down at once. Learn to eat slowly and don't be afraid to save some for later.

4. **Enough with the booze.** There are lots of reasons why drinking isn't good for you. Like fast food, we all know about them, so I won't bother repeating them.

   Tip: Drinking is like everything else on this list—you don't have to give it up completely. Moderation is key; take the amount that you drink now and halve it. If you can stick to this new schedule, it will help your fitness level considerably. When you're out with friends, try alternating an alcoholic drink with a glass of water. This will lessen the amount that you drink, save you money, make you feel better in the morning and most of all, still allow you to have something in your hand so that you don't feel awkward or uncomfortable in a crowded bar.

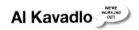
5. **Cut out soda and other sugary drinks.** Lots of people don't seem to realize how bad soda is for you. It's packed with sugar (or worse!) and a surprising number of calories. One 12-ounce can of soda can have up to 200 calories. The beverage world can be tricky. Vitamin Water, for example, is not good for you. Even though its title implies healthiness, it's really almost as bad as most sodas. As a general rule, if something tastes overly sweet and delicious, chances are it's loaded with sugar and not good for you.

   Tip: Drink water. It's refreshing and has no calories. If this gets too bland for you, add a twist of lemon or change it up by getting an unsweetened iced tea. Don't bother trying to fool your taste buds with diet sodas—they're loaded with chemicals! At first this might be tough, but your taste buds will adapt to having less sugar and you'll come to appreciate how good it can feel to have a refreshing glass of water.

6. **Pay Attention.** This is both the simplest and the most complicated rule to follow. Pay attention while you're eating and make a conscious effort to eat a little slower. That doesn't sound so hard, right? Here's another important one: when you feel full, stop eating. Both of these practices are easier to understand than to implement. This is where mindfulness comes in to play. Distraction doesn't just happen during your workout. Take accountability in the moment. Oh, and don't super-size. I mean, come on.

   Tip: Restaurants give you too much food and fast food joints practically throw calories in your face. Consider saving half of your meal for lunch the next day. If you take your time and try to appreciate each bite, you might find that you're actually full before you're done.

In short, just try to eat smart and don't get discouraged. If you go out one night to some fancy place and get the two pound T-bone with creamy mashed potatoes and a bottle of wine, or you find yourself late night ordering a double cheeseburger at some trashy fast food place, don't worry about it and don't beat yourself up over it. Instead, wake up the next day and get back to your plan. So many people who fail at getting fit do so because they believe in the all-or-nothing principle: if they can't stick to their diet 24/7 and adhere exactly to their fitness regimen, they believe that it is not worth doing at all and give up. That's the real mistake, giving up.

You should approach your diet from a day-to-day viewpoint. If you can keep yourself from getting that big, greasy cheeseburger today, you win. If you order a side of vegetables instead of mac and cheese, you win. Don't worry about tomorrow until tomorrow. Take each day as it comes and try to win every day. Keep your mind and your focus in the present and concentrate on what you're doing now. If you can manage to do this and not worry about the future, you'll be pleasantly surprised by what the future brings.

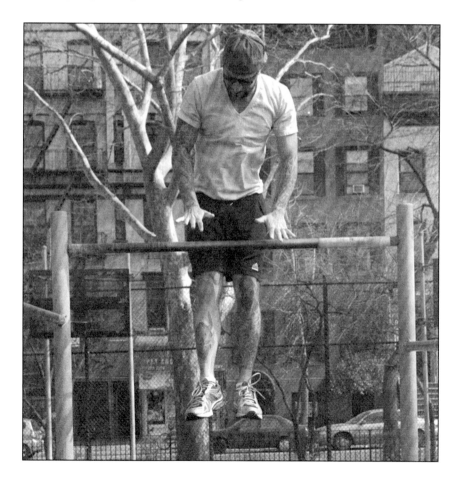

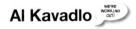

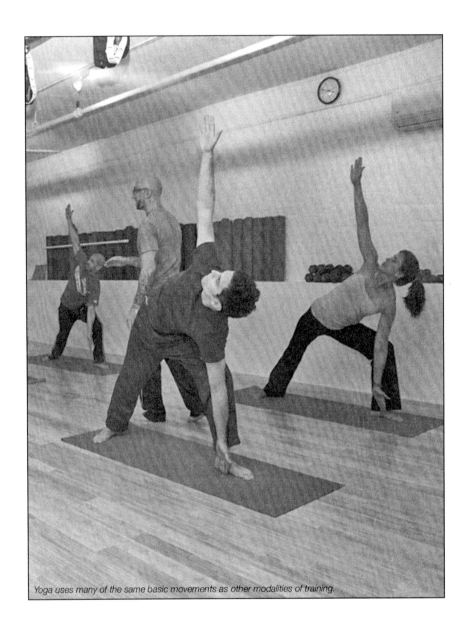

Yoga uses many of the same basic movements as other modalities of training.

Chapter Two:
Exercising (and) Mindfulness

This might sound a bit odd, but the type of exercise that you do isn't all that important. Whether it's push-ups in your house and running around the block, or rock climbing and playing tennis—it doesn't matter, as long as you're working smartly, safely and efficiently. The old saying goes, "Don't work harder, work smarter," but I disagree. I say, "Work hard AND work smart."

Let's start with working smart. What does this mean? Mindfulness is at the center of my fitness philosophy and it's the belief from which all of my practices are born. In its most basic sense, mindfulness means that your attention is entirely focused on the task that you are performing at a particular moment. In short, paying attention to what you're doing when you're doing it. If, as you read this, you get distracted by another thought (maybe your mom's birthday is next week and you haven't figured out what to get her…flowers, maybe?) then you are NOT exercising mindfulness. If you're reading a book, read the book. If you're thinking about what to get Mom, think about what to get Mom. And if you're exercising, think about exercising.

Exercising mindfully means that during your workout you are concentrating on the present moment and not drifting off into a daydream or worrying about what you will do next. Before beginning your routine, try to let go of the clutter occupying your mental space. If you're frustrated at work or you had a fight with your girlfriend, don't take that anxiety and confusion into your workout. Take a moment

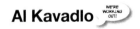

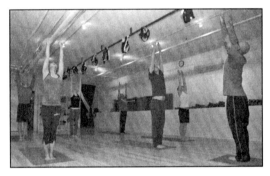

beforehand to relax yourself and slow your mind. This might be hard at first, but with time and practice you will be able to clear your mind and focus on the task at hand. When you learn to improve your concentration, you will improve your workout. Just bear in mind that this is going to be a slow process.

I think it's safe to assume that most people reading this book have attempted some form of organized exercise at least once in their life. Perhaps you found it to be agony, the burning in your lungs too much to bear, the aching in your legs insufferable. Or maybe you liked it, but were unable to keep up with your regimen. No matter your viewpoint, there were probably times when you had a hard time keeping focused. It's pretty common. Anyone who exercises, no matter how long they have been at it, will sometimes drift off during a workout. A catchy tune on your iPod or the person running on the treadmill next to you can throw you out of your rhythm and take over your mind in a fraction of a second. We see this in our everyday lives, as well. Whether you're at the gym, at work, reading a book or driving a car, distractions will happen. And guess what? That's fine. When you feel yourself drifting, bring your focus back to the task at hand, whether it is pull-ups or just keeping the car on the road.

There are certain activities like driving or operating heavy machinery that we as a society deem more attention worthy than others. Generally, these are actions that require increased concentration and focus in order to maintain safety, and with good reason. We all know the dangers involved when people become distracted behind the wheel. You catch your reflection in the rearview mirror and wonder if that zit is still going to be there for your date on Saturday and then wham! You slam into the car in front of you. If you lose your attention for even a moment, the consequences can be tragic. It's with this mindset that I want you to go into every workout. This is mindfulness.

The way I see it, being behind the wheel of an automobile is no more important of an undertaking than being "behind the wheel" of your own body. You should take the same care and precaution in your workout as you do with staying on the road (there are lots of terrible drivers out there, too, but I digress). Unfortunately, most people don't share my point of view and fail to take their workouts very seriously. To them, exercise is a pain in the ass, something to get done with as soon as possible so that they can get back to their lives. They even go so far as to intentionally distract themselves while exercising. All of the gyms in America's major cities are now equipped with rows and rows of TVs in order to cater to this need for distraction. People watch the TVs so that they won't have to think about what they're doing, about the stress that their bodies are going through. If they can just make it through that episode of *Everybody Loves Raymond*, they can throw in the towel and go home feeling good about themselves. It is this distractionary approach to exercise, this reliance on a diverted mind, which I am trying to prevent.

Let's go back to the car metaphor for a minute. If you're driving along on the highway and talking on your cell phone, you're more likely to get in an accident. "But I've done this before," you say. "I'm not going to drive off the road." And this is probably true, but while your attention is diverted, you're missing other things that are just as important. The speed limit is 65, but you glance down after a couple minutes and realize you're going 90. You back off a bit, but then get sucked back into your phone call. By the time you glance back down, you're going 40 and cars are flying past you. Your equilibrium is off and you're unable to maintain that 60-miles-per-hour limit.

While driving a car is clearly more dangerous than going for a run (you're less likely to injure others while working out), your body works in the same way. If your attention is focused on something else, you might miss the signs that your body is sending you. While you're chatting away, clues that you should be speeding up or slowing down are slipping by you like cars on the highway. When you're working out, you should be constantly listening to your body. Not only will this improve your workout from day to day, it will also help you to avoid injury.

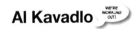
Al Kavadlo

Now you might be saying, "But I hate working out. Why would I want to think about that the whole time? It will just make me hate it more." I understand this—it makes sense. If something is making you miserable, why harp on it? Why channel all your energy and attention into it? I can answer these questions with the same points that I brought up earlier (because you'll get a better workout, because otherwise you might get hurt, etc.), but I can also answer them in another way, one that you might not have expected. Ready for it?

BECAUSE YOU MIGHT JUST START TO LIKE IT.

Seems crazy, right? Well, humans are an extremely adaptable species. Think about it. There are people simultaneously living in Alaska while others are living in rainforests. One group ended up in the north and learned to survive in the frigid cold; the other went to the forests and learned to live a life amongst the trees and humidity. Both groups had to adapt to survive. While your circumstances might not be as dire as these, the fact still remains that your body is wired to adapt.

Need a different example? A more familiar one? Fine. Think about the first time you had a beer. Do you remember what that was like? It was bitter and gross. If your friends hadn't all been standing around, you probably would have spit it out. Now, years later, a cold beer can be refreshing and enjoyable. Over time, your body adapted to the taste of beer and your mind stopped associating it with bitterness and began associating it with more pleasant effects (getting buzzed). So what's my point? It can be the same with exercise. Right now, you dread it because it tires you out and burns your muscles. Your mind focuses on the negative aspects, the bitterness. What you need to do is start to slowly change your mindset and the best way to do this is NOT by watching TV and ignoring what you're doing! It's focusing on your workout while you're doing it. It's getting into the exercises and being involved. It's listening to what your body is telling you. It's exercising mindfulness. Before you know it, exercise might be as refreshing and enjoyable as a cold beer.

PLANNING YOUR WORKOUT

My clients always ask me about what kind of regimen they should be following. What's the best method? What should they do each day? How much time should they be spending? My answer is always the same: listen to your body.

One of the main reasons why it is essential to be in tune with your body during your workout is so you can effectively gauge how much you can handle on any given day. Some people enter the gym with a preconceived plan of what they want to do that day. This is a great idea, but you must also be ready to make spontaneous adjustments based on what your body is telling you. If you are watching TV or too concerned with being seen at the gym (or seeing others), you may be missing the big picture. Sometimes listening to your body will mean you won't push yourself as hard as you may have planned, but, more often than not, we tend to sell ourselves short and stop before we have pushed ourselves to what our bodies can handle.

Others go into the gym without much of a plan at all. They wander about aimlessly, eventually winding up in the hot tub or sauna, as if just being in the gym is going to get them fit. Obviously, this isn't ideal either. It's best to aim for the middle ground between being too regimented and being totally unstructured.

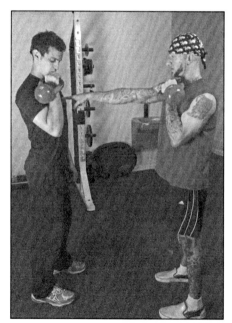

When developing your workout routine, it is best to seek guidance from others. Like with all things in life, however, only take the advice that works for you and makes sense to you. While it's great to get ideas from others who have been down the road before you, remember that each journey is unique and you must find the path for yourself. Listen to what others have to say, but also learn to trust your instincts. Once again, pay attention to how your body reacts. If someone suggests an exercise that doesn't feel right to you, then change it or try a different exercise altogether. No two bodies are exactly alike, so your exercises shouldn't be either.

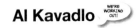

Al Kavadlo

The best people to help design workouts are personal trainers simply because they have the experience. You can use their knowledge to find what works for you and what will help your body the most. When I started training, I used to really stress out about setting up a program for my clients. During each session, I would stand there with a clipboard that had all the exercises I had planned for that client. This might be helpful for new trainers because it makes them feel more organized and in control. However, as I became more experienced, I realized that half the time I'd have to change my plan anyway. If a client had played basketball the day before and wrenched his shoulder a little or overworked a particular muscle group, it might cancel out half the exercises I had planned for him. As a result, I'd have to come up with new ones on the spot, which was even more stressful. Eventually, I ditched the clipboard and started my sessions with only a general plan in mind, one that allowed for change and adaptability and put less stress on my client and myself. When planning your own workout, keep this experience in mind. Come up with a basic regimen, but don't feel like you need to stick to it letter for letter. Adapting is a good thing. If you alter your workout slightly because of something you feel, it means you're listening to your body and acting on what it's telling you. It means you're being mindful and that's good.

Try to keep in mind, however, that trainers aren't always right and advice isn't always helpful. Don't be afraid to question authority (even mine) and remember that no one has all the answers, no matter their level of qualification. Also, no one knows your body better than you do, so don't be afraid to ask questions and make a trainer earn your trust. While a trainer may have lots of experience, it is important for them to keep an open mind when it comes to your training program: both you and your trainer should try to maintain the beginner's mind. This might be a little confusing to you, so I'll try to clarify it through the words of Shunryu Suzuki in his work *Zen Mind, Beginner's Mind*. He says, "In the mind of the beginner there are many possibilities, in the mind of the expert there are few."

I think what Suzuki is saying here is when we think we know everything, we look at the world through a narrower scope. We think we've seen it all and heard it all already, so we find a way to reject whatever isn't within that small spectrum of vision. We lose the ability to learn and grow. We also can lose our appreciation for the beauty of simple, everyday things. It's kind of like what we often call "taking things for granted," which is something far too many of us do (myself included). As a result, it is important to approach each moment (or for our concerns, each workout) with an open mind and a fresh perspective. One ought to stay present and not assume that things will happen a certain way simply because they have played out that way before. On the other side of the coin, having experience helps to improve one's ability to make adjustments when the need to do so presents itself. Perhaps what we need experience in is the very act of being in the now.

The more you think you know, the harder it is to learn something new. Even as a trainer, it is important for me to keep my mind open to all possibilities and listen to my client. By following this practice, I've learned a lot from the people I've trained. They've asked questions I hadn't considered, pointed out problems that I had overlooked and even helped me discover ways to improve myself. This is the ideal relationship between trainer and client; your training should be a give and take process that enlightens you both.

EVALUATING YOUR WORKOUT

People often ask me how they can judge the effectiveness of their workout. Usually they're looking for me to tell them an ideal heart rate range, how fast they should run or how much weight they should be lifting (we all love to be evaluated and told that we are doing well). While these are all effective ways of measuring a workout, the best way to answer these questions is not with a statistic, but rather by examining how you feel. As I hinted at before, there are so many factors that can change on a day-to-day basis that a plan you have on Sunday may not be reasonable to follow come Monday. The amount of sleep you have had, what you ate and everything that has happened in your day can affect the quality of your workout. The best way to gauge the effectiveness of your workout is to feel the effects of it. Be there for every moment of the workout and push yourself hard.

Here is what I want you to try. The next time you are working out, focus all of your attention on whatever you are doing in that moment. If you are warming up, then just warm up. Try not to think too much about the next step; instead, think about the step you are taking now. If you are lifting weights, focus on controlling your

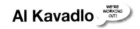
movement and getting the best contraction possible out of each rep. If you are running, feel your foot hit the ground on every stride. Feel your knees bend and your hip extending as you push into your next stride. While exercising, you will inevitably be bombarded with a barrage of thoughts and stimuli, which will make it hard to keep your focus. This is sometimes known as "Monkey Mind"—you jump around from thought to thought like a monkey jumps from tree to tree. You're all over the place! This is okay. Simply bring your attention back to your breathing and begin again. Try to train your monkey to sit still for a bit. Allow him to rest in one tree, while you move on with your workout. He's an excitable monkey though, so you're likely to repeat this cycle over and over as you're working out. Don't panic, you're not doing anything wrong. Becoming distracted by your thoughts is natural and can't be completely avoided. The important thing is to bring your mind back into focus. You might be surprised by how difficult this actually is, but don't try to assess how well you are doing it, simply do it.

Staying in the present moment can seem frustrating, pointless or even impossible to many people at first; our brains have become so deeply conditioned to relying on distractions. Even with much practice, there will be times when you'll become discouraged. When this happens, try to keep in mind that some days are simply going to be harder than others and that's okay. I've had workouts where I just can't help but think about whatever is stressing me out. I can't keep myself from having these thoughts, so it does me no good to do anything other than let them pass. Then I bring my attention back to the task at hand. You will never be able to fully quiet your thoughts, so don't be frustrated when you can't. This is not a technique that can be mastered, it's merely an exercise that can help you to temporarily clear the clutter in your mind. Achieving that calm for even a few seconds is an accomplishment—its fleeting nature should not be taken with frustration, but with fulfillment. Just those few seconds of peace can help center you and heighten your awareness.

Think about it like visiting the Grand Canyon on an overcast day. When you first arrive, a heavy fog has settled in and the canyon is blocked completely from view. As you stand there annoyed and squinty-eyed, sunlight suddenly breaks through the clouds, illuminating the entire canyon. For several seconds you can take in the canyon's full glory. Then, just as quickly as it vanished, the fog returns, once again removing the canyon from sight. Naturally, you might be a little frustrated at having lost such a beautiful sight so quickly, but would it be better to have never seen it at all, to have gone home having missed the canyon completely? Of course not. You got a glimpse, even if only for a moment. When you can dissipate the fog in your mind and clear the clouds for a few seconds, appreciate the experience. Concentrate on the view, not the brevity. Your greatest and most effective workouts can be when you're nearing the edge of the canyon, waiting for the view to clear.

Now it's a cliché, but I'm going to say it anyway: anything that's worth doing is going to be difficult, especially at first. Finding your calm is not easy; anyone who says otherwise is lying. It takes time and patience. It can't happen in one afternoon or during a weekend retreat, even if you pay hundreds of dollars to some "Zen Master." The key is to get yourself into a mindset where you are not concerned with the end result. Staying the course over a long period of time is a daunting prospect. If you're only focused on a goal and how long it will take to get there, you'll inevitably begin to feel overwhelmed. Constantly worrying about the future and "how you're progressing," can weigh down your mind and hold you back. It's much simpler and more practical to simply focus on what you are doing now and doing it as best as you can. Focus on that every time, and that is all you will ever need to be concerned about. And don't worry, progress will come and it will show.

ENJOYMENT

One of the main tenets of my exercise philosophy is that enjoyment is essential to success. To put it simply, if you continue to hate working out, you're not going to last. I'm sorry, but that's the truth. You might stick with it for a couple weeks or even a month or two, but if you can't find a way to enjoy it, you're doomed. The key is to find an activity that appeals to you.

There are hundreds of ways to exercise and if you try enough options, chances are you will find something that you like enough to make it a priority. One of the cool things about my personal journey is that through my obsession with getting the "perfect six-pack" (I'll get to this in a minute), I discovered things that I probably wouldn't have otherwise tried. One of those things was running, which despite

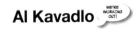
hating at first, I grew to truly love and appreciate. Running is something that I make time to do at least once or twice a week no matter what other exercise program I might be doing. I think running is something everyone should try. It's the most natural and easy way to get fit and it's totally free. Just go outside and start running. Even if you hate it at first, like I did, give it a couple weeks and see if you change your mind. As your body adapts to running and you get into something of a habit, your perception of it will change and you might just start to love it.

Running works for me and makes up a good portion of my exercise regimen, but if it doesn't work for you, that's fine. Like I said, there are plenty of other options. When I first started working out, I stuck mainly to weight training. Lifting was what I knew best and gave me a certain level of comfort and confidence, but over the years I have expanded my repertoire considerably. I've included calisthenics, running, cycling, yoga, martial arts, rock climbing, tennis, kayaking and whatever else strikes my fancy. I point this out because I often hear friends and clients tell me that they stopped working out because they got sick of their routine. It's all I can do to keep from yelling, "So change it! Don't give up!" If you're ever losing interest in your workout, start trying new things, new ways to get out and be active. If you're tired of running, try rounding up some friends to play basketball. If you've had enough of yoga, try swimming. If you're sick of the gym, grab a buddy and bang a ball around your local tennis court. Whether it's running, skiing or simply doing jumping jacks in your room, it doesn't matter. As long as you're working your body in an effective and safe way, then you're making progress. Boredom is not an excuse for laziness. Don't quit simply because an exercise is starting to get a little stale. With that said, don't ignore your fading interest either, listen to it. Exercise routines, like many of life's routines, will inevitably become dull when they are repeated over and over again. And this isn't just a mental thing; your body also gets bored when you repeat the same action. When you have the combined effect of both your body and your mind losing interest, you'll end up in a rut or you'll hit a plateau.

Remember, fitness is something you'll be doing for the rest of your life. Sound scary? It shouldn't, and when you start enjoying your workouts, it won't seem so daunting. What if I told you you'd have to eat ice cream every day for the rest of your life? That wouldn't be so bad, right? Once you can find a way to enjoy fitness, the idea of doing it every day won't seem so overwhelming. Find a way to continuously immerse yourself in various activities and you'll likely begin to have fun with the process. Once you learn to enjoy your workout, you won't have to worry about forcing yourself to go to the gym. You'll be happy to go and that makes all the difference.

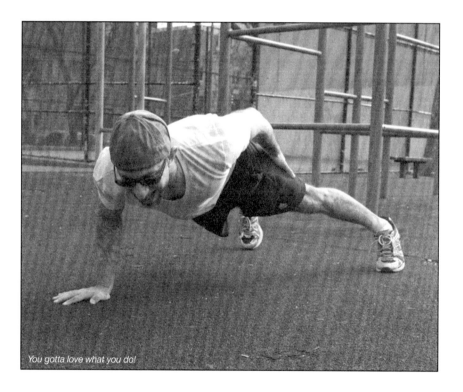

You gotta love what you do!

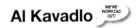

Chapter Three:
Breathe

The simple act of breathing is one of the most miraculous things our bodies do and yet we hardly notice it. It's among the most fundamental processes that keep us alive and it happens without any effort. In meditation, which exercise can be a form of, attention to your breath is one of the most frequently taught practices. Controlled breathing increases focus and calms the mind. Your breath is like an anchor in a sea of churning thoughts. If you can use it as such, you will improve not only your workouts, but also your concentration in general.

In most modalities of training, it is common to pay attention to your breathing and there is usually a technique involved with it. In weight training, we emphasize inhaling when lowering the weight and exhaling when lifting. The idea is that having your breath behind you when pushing allows for greater force production. In some schools of yoga, the Ujjayi breathing technique is taught. Ujjayi breathing enables the practitioner to maintain energy and focus during yoga practice, while simultaneously helping to clear toxins out of the body. Similarly, most serious runners are aware of the way their breath syncs up with their pacing and the movement of their legs. Taking this approach and using efficient, controlled breathing makes their workouts as effective as possible. Perhaps more importantly, practicing any of these techniques allows the breath itself to function as a means of keeping your attention on the present moment.

When I say, "Concentrate on your breathing," people are often confused as to what I really mean. This is tough to explain because different types of training call for different breathing techniques. The best way to help you understand is by leading you through a brief and basic breathing exercise. It's very simple and you can do it right now. Read the steps below and then put the book down and try it. Ready?

Step 1. Breathe in through your nose, slowly, but deeply and completely. Feel your lungs fill up and your chest expand. Notice your back straighten. Keep going until your lungs are completely full and you can't breathe in any more.

Step 2. Breathe out through your mouth slowly. Keep pushing your breath past where you normally would and empty your lungs completely. Push the air out until there's nothing left to push, then push a little more. Feel it as it leaves, as your chest and diaphragm constrict, tightening your core.

Step 3. Breathe in again and repeat the first two steps.

After doing this a few times, do you feel calmer? Looser? Notice how really thinking about the process of fully breathing in and out makes your mind block out all other

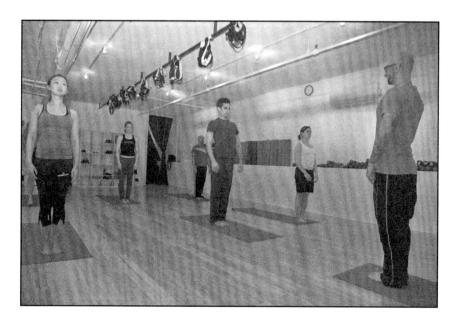

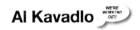

distractions. You are so focused on that single act that all the white noise and whirring thoughts fade into the background and you are calmed. This feeling will go away and your calm will pass, but remember what it feels like and take a moment every once in a while to come back to it.

Concentrating on your breathing before a workout can help you focus as you begin. As you start your exercise, try to pay attention to the way your body naturally breathes; don't do anything, just observe. As you run, your breath will become more rapid on its own. Don't mess with the rhythm, just focus on it as it goes in and out and matches up with your stride. As you continue, try to maintain this focus. If you get distracted, and you will at times, just take a deep breath and start over. This process is difficult and takes some time to get the hang of, but when you can reach that state of calm, it is worth it.

MINDFULNESS VS. GOALS

The practice of mindfulness is often associated with Zen, a component of Buddhism. Now don't worry, I am not going to get all religious on you, that's not what this book is about. The way I approach Zen is more of a philosophy than a religion. To me, Zen is simply taking the most direct approach to dealing with your life and your surroundings. I'll be frank with you; I've never been to Tibet to study with the monks. I'm not really well traveled at all, actually, having spent most of my life in New York. A lot of people might say that I don't know anything about true Zen and perhaps they're right. So feel free to call me a big phony if you want. I'll tell you this much though, there is no faking it when it comes to your body. If you don't feel like you've truly tapped into your life's potential, then you owe it to yourself to rectify the situation. Don't allow that yearning to go ignored.

Different people come to discover mindfulness and Zen in different ways— meditation, martial arts or even motorcycle maintenance. Others, like me, find it through exercise. Regardless of the style, each method is simply a doorway that leads to the same thing. We are each trying to grasp a small piece of that wisdom through uniting our bodies and minds.

In Buddhism, there are Four Noble Truths that make up the backbone of the religion. The first is usually translated as, "Life is suffering." Yikes. I know, it sounds pretty brutal. To me though, it simply means that life ain't easy. No matter what you do, there will always be something about life that isn't quite perfect. Even if you get it perfect for one moment, that moment will inevitably pass. We can never have all of our desires fulfilled, but learning to accept this makes more sense than trying to change it.

Buddha says attachment is the root of all suffering. If we stop focusing on the desire to reach a goal and savor the moment instead, we can begin to alleviate this suffering. This is where Zen and mindfulness come in to the picture.

Zen is a way in which to deal with life. It utilizes mindfulness meditation as a way to get the most out of every day—to truly see life for what it is. In other words, mindfulness is therapeutic. By practicing it, you can't remove the day's suffering (whether it be a family tragedy or simply a bad day at work), but you can deal with what you're doing **now**. If you can enter your workout with that mindset, you're already ahead of the game.

When exercising, it is important to remain focused, yet relaxed. Mental clutter gets in the way of your concentration and breaks your focus. The best athletes are able to shut out the roar of the crowd and the pressure of the big game. When a basketball player is standing at the foul line and needs to make a free throw to win the game, he isn't focusing on the fans that are screaming and waving flashy objects behind the basket. He's focusing on staying calm, setting his feet and making the basket. Being able to shut out excess stimuli is often the key to success. Next time you're watching a game, look at the player's face as he's setting up his shot. I bet you he takes a few controlled breaths before he releases the ball.

In Zazen (formal seated meditation), there is no activity other than sitting and breathing. The mind has very little stimulation, which can be quite jarring to how our brains have become conditioned. The mindfulness practiced during exercise, however, goes in a different direction than pure mindfulness meditation. You are trying to be mindful while performing a task (more like the basketball player than a monk). That said, if you're interested in meditation and Zen outside of your workouts, I encourage you to look into them more deeply. Freeing yourself further from the constraints of your mind might help improve your workouts. However, your

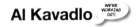

experience is unique to you, while mine is unique to me. Since your ideas about Zen, spirituality, religion, etc. might be different than mine, you should feel free to add to or modify my suggestions to make them a better fit for you. That's the beauty of exercising and fitness. It's all about you.

A big part of the mindfulness philosophy is attempting to free yourself from judgment. Try to avoid putting things into categories of right and wrong or good and bad. Don't judge your workout as good or bad and don't judge your mindfulness practice as good or bad. However, it is okay if you have these thoughts, just try not to judge yourself for having them.

In Zen, it is said that there is no doing something right, there is only doing something. Of course, this gets a little tricky when it comes to exercise. Most people view exercise in terms of goals. Their goal may be to lose weight, improve stamina or gain muscle. It is how Americans are conditioned to think. Mindfulness is not concerned with goals; it is concerned with the present moment. This doesn't mean that you can't achieve a goal while practicing mindfulness. It might seem like the two are at odds with one another, but that is not so.

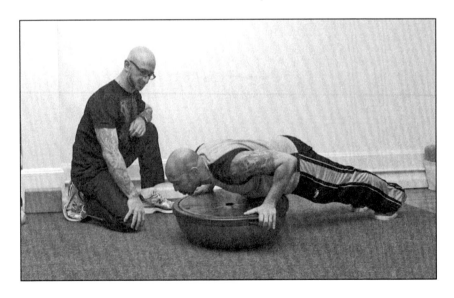

A WATCHED POT

You've probably heard the expression, "A watched pot never boils." The lesson is pretty simple—patience. Staring at a pot and willing it to boil won't affect the rate at which it boils. Rushing and focusing on the end result will only frustrate you, but if you relax and don't worry about the water, it will be boiling before you know it. Keep this lesson in mind when thinking about your fitness goals.

People who are overly concerned about their progress and achieving their fitness goals might feel the need to check if their time spent exercising and dieting is working. Every day they jump on the scale, checking their progress. Some people will let their entire day be colored by what the scale tells them in the morning. Improved fitness is a gradual process and it's unlikely that people will see any significant change in a short amount of time. Such frequent "watching the pot" can be disheartening and lead to frustration. Instead of scale watching and mirror checking, try to concern yourself only with the process. If you're not worried about how close you are to your goal, then you're more likely to stick with your program. I know the idea of no goal sounds strange; it's the opposite of how we usually think, but it's the process that matters. If you continue working and focusing on what you're doing, you'll find that others will notice changes, whether you can see them yet or not. Be patient. Your water will boil.

THE IDEA OF SUCCESS

Mindfulness and patience are not easily achieved. I've never been one hundred percent happy with the way that my body looks. I don't know if anybody is. For a long time, the area that bothered me most was my abdomen. What drove me crazy was that I could never seem to achieve what I thought was the "perfect six-pack." I tried so many different routines for working my abs over the years, each time thinking, "This is the one!" Inevitably, about three months into each program, I would stand in front of my mirror and try to figure out if I could see any difference. There would be some changes here and there, but I never reached a point where I was satisfied. I wanted perfection, but it kept eluding me. I kept my diets impeccably clean and healthy for months and concentrated all my energy on working my abs and my core. It was starting to verge on an unhealthy obsession, and I still couldn't get the look I wanted.

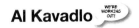
I know this sounds like something you might hear at the start of some infomercial for a new fitness product like the Ab-o-matic or the Tummy Titan 2000, but this story doesn't end with me finding the perfect exercise or the miracle product. As it turns out, I never got the Brad Pitt abs I wanted. Instead, having recently started practicing mindfulness and meditation, I began to change my perception of myself. Focusing on the process and taking a step back from my goal completely changed my understanding of my body. Years later, I feel much better about my body, even though I don't really look much different. This shift in perspective happened gradually as I tried workout after workout and kept ending up with the same result. Eventually, I was able to accept the truth and stop denying the obvious reality: the "problem" with my abs wasn't within my abdomen, but within my mind.

Now you might be thinking that I gave up on my fitness goal, that I failed, but I can assure you I didn't. I train harder and with more passion than ever before, the change is that I don't obsess over minor "flaws" that I can't do anything about. The more I focus on the workout itself and the less I focus on the outcome, the more I enjoy everything about the process, including the outcome. My body looks better to me now than it ever did when I was focused on the results.

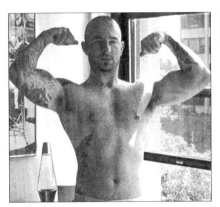 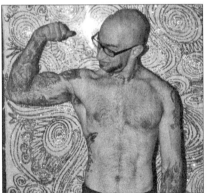

Left: I was never satisfied with the results when I was trying to look like a bodybuilder. (2003) Right: I still don't have a perfect six-pack but I love my body and I feel amazing! (2010)

Chapter Four:
Why Bother?

Whenever I talk about my program, people want to know what they'll get out of it. They can't help but ask, "Why, why, why?"

Why should I do this?

Why should I give all this effort and dedicate all this time?

Why not do something quick and easy?

These are all fair questions and I'll go through each, but you might be surprised by how much you already know.

WHY SHOULD I DO THIS?

If you're not currently working out or you're being lazy about it, there are plenty of obvious reasons to start or amp up your regimen. You've heard them all before, but they are important, so let's go through them. The most important reason is your health. Heart disease is the number one cause of death in the United States. It ranks higher than cancer, influenza and traffic accidents. All the crap that we eat, combined with the stress of our everyday lives and our sedentary lifestyle, is literally killing us. Every doughnut you devour while sitting on your couch, every nacho you drizzle with cheese while watching the game and every super-sized meal you inhale on your way back from a stressed out day at the office; they're all taking shots at your heart—a collection of jabs and uppercuts that are beating your poor heart to a pulp. Our hearts aren't punching bags. They just can't take that kind of abuse.

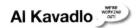
Al Kavadlo

I know that's a little depressing, but the news isn't all bad. You can change this downward spiral and start to reverse the damage. You just need to get off your ass and be a little more mindful of your lifestyle and what it's doing to your body. You only have one body, and it's all you're going to get so start taking action. Of course, that's the hardest part—getting yourself up and moving. Despite being a personal trainer, I occasionally have this problem, but I've found a system that helps me overcome it. (By the way, some of the laziest people I know are trainers. It's hard for everyone!)

When I'm tired, hung-over or just plain worn out, the gym is often the last place I feel like going. But, like I said earlier, once I get there and through my workout, I'm ALWAYS happy I did it. I feel better, more energized and more productive. Of course, that doesn't make getting there any easier. So how do I do it? Just like with exercising itself, I concentrate on the present. When I wake up, I don't think about how bad the workout is going to be or how much my head is going to hurt when I'm running. In fact, I don't think about the workout at all. I simply concentrate on getting out of bed.

I aim to handle each little morning task on its own. While I'm brushing my teeth, I'm only thinking about brushing my teeth. Then I'll put my clothes on, drink some water, eat some breakfast and do whatever else I need to do before heading to work out. The key is to take things one at a time, step by step. Why worry about the gym when I can be enjoying my breakfast? Stay in the present. Just like I suggested that you try not to think about your day-to-day stresses during your workout, I advise you not to think too much about your workout when you are dealing with your day-to-day life. This can be hard, naturally, so if you can't help yourself from thinking about the future, simply try to focus on how good you are going to feel after you push yourself through your routine. Be positive—you can do this. Remember all those other people that get it done…is it any easier for them? C'mon now!

WHY SHOULD I GIVE ALL THIS EFFORT AND DEDICATE ALL THIS TIME?
For most of us, our personal image is directly related to our self-esteem. When we know that we've been letting ourselves go a little, it affects how we feel. Vanity

shouldn't be your main motivation, but if it gives you the impetus to get going, that isn't a bad thing. When you see a change in your body, it can certainly be uplifting, but often we get too carried away with appearances. Your happiness should not be contingent upon what you see in the mirror.

I mentioned earlier that we are an extremely adaptable species, but what I didn't mention is that there's a downside to this. We can adapt to the toughest of circumstances, but we can also adapt to the easiest. Just as exercise can become addicting, so can inactivity. If you're always inactive, your body and your mind will start to identify that as your normal state. Once your brain gets into this habit, it will attempt to maintain it because it has identified it as "good." Sitting on the couch feels good and working out doesn't, so your adaptive brain will encourage you to remain inactive. This is trouble! Even though your brain has declared this state as comfortable and seeks to maintain it, you're more likely to become depressed and unhealthy. Fortunately, since you're adaptable, you can break this habit and retrain your brain. I know this sounds a little weird, but once you start exercising, your brain begins firing in new ways. It will release endorphins and start associating exercise and activity with feeling good. When you're trying to overcome your laziness, remember that our bodies aren't designed to just sit around. We're hunters and gatherers—we're supposed to be moving! Immobility isn't natural; your body had to be taught how to be lazy.

Don't believe me? Think about kids. To a child, sitting still is like torture, all they ever want to do is run around and play. They run until they are exhausted, until they can barely keep their eyes open, but they love every second of it. Next time you're laying around, think of your six-year-old self and what he or she would say if they saw you sitting there. "Come on, play with me!" Don't fight that urge, embrace it.

WHY NOT DO SOMETHING QUICK AND EASY?
I've made it clear that I don't really care what exercise program(s) you decide to use. There are plenty of serious ones out there and the key is to find what works for you. What I am hoping to do is empower you. I am here to show you that if you really want to get stronger, lose weight, build muscle and improve your fitness level (or your life!), you can. All you have to do is take action.

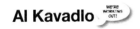

There are good programs out there, but there are also a lot of not-so-good ones. In my opinion, anything that encourages spending as little time as possible is not a great program. If an ad says you only need to exercise for seven minutes every day, I say that's ridiculous! If you're serious about getting in shape, you must push the envelope a little. Don't allow yourself to be limited by what other people (especially people selling something) tell you. Listen to your body and act accordingly. That said, a few minutes a day isn't bad for you. It's not ideal, but it's still better than nothing. The movement from nothing to something is the biggest step. Once the ball is rolling, you can start to pick up some momentum.

I think a word of warning is necessary here. When choosing a workout program, don't be foolish. There are no magic pills that will make you lose weight without exercising and there are no vibrating machines that will burn fat and trim your body while you sit around. Of course, these kinds of products can seem tempting when you're feeling tired or desperate, but don't fall for them. They are gimmicks designed to play on the hopes of the lazy and emotionally vulnerable. Don't let yourself be fooled. Deep down, you know that these products won't work, so save your money and start making a conscious effort to change yourself.

As I've said, my philosophy is a no-nonsense approach to getting fit. The reason to follow my method is simply because it makes sense. Don't use a program that encourages you to slack off and take the easy route. Instead, embrace your urge to better yourself and then immerse yourself in the process of doing just that. Nothing worth doing is easy, but challenges are what make life exciting!

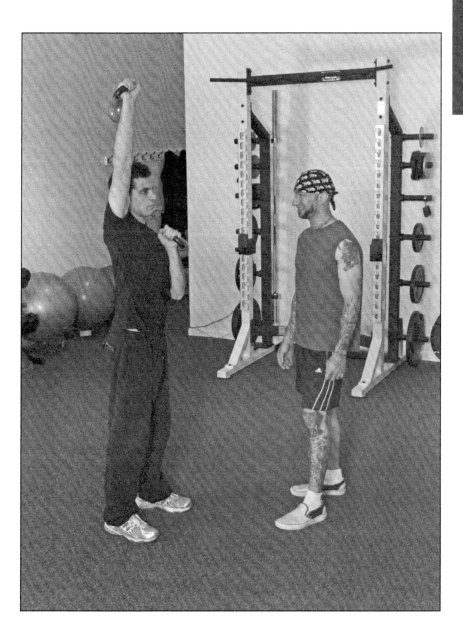

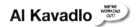

Chapter Five:
My Top Five

When I tell people that I don't really care what kind of exercises they're doing, as long as they're working hard, it's usually not what they want to hear. They want to know which exercises and what routines I think are the best. Well, there's no such thing as the best exercise, but since everyone always asks for it, I will tell you my favorites (in a second!).

Lots of people (authors, salespeople and even some trainers) will try to sell you the latest "new exercise." In truth though, there aren't really any new exercises. There are thousands of different ways to work out, but when you break them down, they're really just new ways to do the same old thing. Everything else is just a makeover, new packaging on an old product to make it seem more enticing. That's why cola companies change their cans all the time. The recipe is still the same—pure sugar—but the new design catches people's eyes and ropes them back for more. However, when it comes to exercise, change is a good thing—variety keeps things from getting stale, but until evolution gives us a third arm or a ball-and-socket joint for a knee, the fundamentals will always stay the same. The subtle variations are infinite, but the basic movements are few. There are really only about a dozen or two basic movements, but I've decided to keep it even simpler than that. If you do these five strength-building basics*, you'll pretty much be set. In fact, I challenge you to do a strength-training workout without incorporating these movements. They come up in everything, including your day-to-day life, so they can't be avoided.

*See appendix for specific routines.

1. PULLING

The pull-up is my all-time favorite exercise. Just like the other workout classics below, the pull-up can be modified in an infinite number of ways. As most of you know from gym class, the basic pull-up works your biceps and the muscles in your back. What a lot of people don't realize is that pull-ups also work your abs, as well as the rest of your body. Technically, a pull-up is done by hanging from an overhead bar with your palms facing away from you. To complete one repetition, pull yourself up until your chin has cleared the bar. Don't limit yourself to just the traditional pull-up, though. Do them with palms facing in (chin-ups) and with palms facing out; do them with a wide grip and a narrow grip and everything in between. The pull-up is a very straightforward exercise, but it's also easily adaptable and extremely effective.

One of my favorite variations is the Australian pull-up. This variant involves hanging below a bar that is set just above waist height, while keeping your heels in contact with the ground. You'll wind up at an angle that is closer to horizontal than vertical. The Australian pull-up is a great way to work up to doing a regular pull-up if you aren't strong enough to do one yet. The Australian pull-up is still worth adding to your routine even if you are strong enough to do lots of regular pull-ups. It puts a little more emphasis on the rear deltoids and the muscles of your middle-back, muscles that may not be getting completely and thoroughly worked with regular pull-ups alone. For those of you who are more advanced, try doing them as a superset, right after a set of regular pull-ups. This is a great way to work towards adding more reps to your pull-up total!

Speaking of the Australian pull-up, rowing movements are another example of upper body pulling. Be it rowing a boat or simulating that movement with a dumbbell or kettlebell (or a machine, I suppose).

Lots of women have trouble with pull-ups when they first start; this is natural. Female bodies are just designed differently. The muscles in that part of their bodies aren't as developed as they are in men. This is not an excuse! I've had many women come up to me and say that pull-ups are impossible for them. Well, guess what? That's garbage. Yes, it will be harder for you to complete a pull-up than it will be for most guys, but that just means you need to work a little harder for it. Take

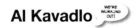

the time and the necessary steps to build muscles in the areas where you're lacking and I promise you will be able to make a pull-up happen.

Also, keep in mind that you don't have to limit yourself to just pull-ups. You can work this same movement with other exercises, too. Pull-downs, for instance, strengthen the same area and are easier to do because the weight is adjustable. A pull-down is usually performed on a machine. Sit down with your back straight, grab the bar (or handles) and simply pull-down. While machines can be a good way to start for some people, I think it's generally better to use your own body weight or free weights to do strength training. That said, pull-downs are still one way to work up to regular pull-ups. But remember, once you can do a pull-up with ease, don't get complacent. When I was starting to feel like I was getting a handle on pull-ups, someone showed me a muscle-up and I was humbled all over again.

A muscle-up begins like a pull-up, but instead of stopping when your chin is over the bar, you continue up until your entire upper body has cleared it. Continually looking for new exercises to try will keep you moving forward and help you continue improving. It will also help you to maintain the beginner's mind.

Trainer Tip: *Pull-ups*—Don't just think about pulling yourself up with your arms. Use your core strength and your entire upper body as you pull your chin over the bar. To help focus and bring everything together, visualize yourself clearing the bar.

2. PUSHING

The push-up is probably the best example of an exercise that requires no equipment. This one exercise alone can make a noticeable change to your chest, shoulders and arms. As I'm sure you all know, to do a basic push-up you start on your hands and toes with a straight line running from your shoulders to your heels. You initiate the movement by lowering yourself to the ground—your chest should touch the ground (or be just an inch above the ground), but your stomach should not. If your stomach is touching the floor, then your form either needs work or you've got a little weight to lose (which is fine!). Make sure you're not sticking your butt in the air either. Focus on keeping your body in a straight line. The movement is about control as much as it is about strength.

If you're having trouble with the basic push-up, you can try keeping your feet on the floor and putting your hands up on a ledge, step or any other sturdy surface that is higher than the floor. This will give you better leverage, making the motion a little easier, but still working the same muscles and allowing you to build up the strength to eventually start regular push-ups. For you more experienced folks, this is a good technique to use while training for one-armed push-ups. By doing a one-armed push-up on an angle, you can get better at the technique and gradually build towards doing them on the floor.

There are endless ways to spice up the push-up. Putting your feet up at an angle against a wall will make them harder because you are putting more weight on your arms. By changing your position, you have less leverage and have to work harder. You can gradually progress to walking your feet all the way up the wall until you wind up doing handstand push-ups! Experiment with different variations of the push-up and it will stay fresh and challenging for you.

The bench press is one of the most popular exercises, but when you think about it, it's basically the same as a push-up…just upside down. Let's break down the movement. There are two things happening when you press the bar away from your chest: your elbows go from bent to straight (the technical name for this is "elbow extension") and your shoulders extend your arms away from your chest (in the world of personal trainers, this is sometimes called "horizontal adduction"). If you break down the push-up, it's exactly the same!

Overhead presses also use the same pushing motion. If you've ever had to lift something heavy over your head, then you've already got some experience with this move. The overhead press is one of the most basic (and functional) exercises out there. Sometimes called a military press or a shoulder press, this exercise has many variations and can be performed with a barbell, dumbbells, kettlebells or any other type of resistance.

The most common way I see people doing overhead presses is with their palms facing forward, away from their body, through the entire range of motion. This is a terrific exercise; however, I am also a big fan of the rotational shoulder press

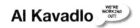
made popular by Arnold Schwarzenegger and often referred to as an Arnold press. This variation involves the palms facing towards the body at the bottom of the movement and rotating outward on the way up. In some cases, the Arnold press can be a safer variation because it provides an increased range of motion without adding stress to your joints.

Dips are another pushing exercise you can do with just your body weight and minimal equipment. Dips involve lowering your body while in an upright position, then pressing back up. If you've never done a dip before, the best way to start is with your feet on the ground and your hands on a ledge or bench. Try not to bend your knees or lose your posture as you lower yourself downward. When your elbows get to a 90 degree angle, push yourself back up and repeat. If you are able to perform more than twenty of these dips with relative ease then you are ready to try dips on parallel bars. A dip station is a pretty standard piece that any gym ought to have. (If your current gym doesn't have a dip station, you might want to start shopping around for a new gym!)

Most men will be able to progress to parallel bar dips relatively quickly. It is generally a much longer process for women, however, due to the fact that women are born with less natural upper body strength than men. This is not me being sexist, ladies—it's just biology!

Trainer Tip: *Push-ups*—Just as with pull-ups, push-ups can be a full body exercise. Keep your legs and core muscles engaged throughout the motion. Think of your body as one unit, rather than as separate parts. If your muscles are working together, you will function more efficiently and your exercise will be more effective.

3. SQUATTING

Squats are probably the single most common exercise I see people needing help with in the gym. Since the movement seems straightforward, most gym-goers think they know how to do a proper squat. The truth is...a lot of them don't know squat!

One of the keys to squatting with safe and effective form is to make sure that you go all the way down until the top of your thigh is parallel to the ground. This might be lower than you think, so try to have someone watch you as you go.

(Please don't crane your neck to look at a mirror, this will throw your spine out of alignment—get a spotter!) Also, keep in mind that your heels should not come off the ground at any point during the lift. The movement should be initiated from the hips, not the knees. What I'm saying is, stick your butt out!

Squats can also be performed on one leg. The most well known type of one-legged squat is the pistol squat, which involves holding your non-squatting leg straight out in front of you. This is a great way to challenge yourself without having to use weights or any equipment. Of course, if you're feeling daring, pistol squats can be done with weight!

While on the subject of squatting, let's not forget about deadlifts. Though deadlifts and squats are technically two different exercises, they are really the same. The big difference between deadlifts and squats is that with deadlifts, you hold the weight in front of you in your hands, instead of resting it on your back or shoulders. Everything else is more or less the same. You puff your chest up, push your heels into the ground and lift the weight.

The two most common types of deadlifts are the Olympic deadlift and the Romanian deadlift. An Olympic deadlift, to put it simply, involves picking up a weight that's on the ground in front of you. I'm sure you've been advised at some point to lift heavy objects with your legs and not your back—that advice is talking about the deadlift! Since it's a motion that you do fairly regularly, this a great functional exercise. This classic version of the deadlift works your lower back and your grip strength more than a squat does. It's also probably the exercise where you'll be able to lift the most weight, just don't get carried away. Remember to lift with your legs, not your ego!

The Romanian deadlift is different than the Olympic deadlift because it involves less knee flexion and more hip flexion. This means that your knees don't bend as much. Instead, you lean over more, sticking your butt out and pushing your chest up and out. If you do a Romanian deadlift with proper form, you should feel a stretch in your hamstrings. It winds up looking more like you're leaning over than sitting down. Romanian deadlifts are great for targeting your butt and hamstrings. This variation is

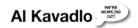
a little less functional than the Olympic deadlift, as you're unlikely to lift an object off the ground like this in everyday life, but it's still beneficial.

For you more advanced folks, consider trying some plyometric jump squats. Plyometric exercises are explosive movements that allow you to take advantage of the elasticity of your muscles—plus jumping is a lot of fun! Make sure whatever you're jumping onto is sturdy, be it a step, a bench or a ledge. To perform the exercise, squat down and then spring up, using your momentum to propel you onto the surface. Land with your knees bent, and then jump back down and repeat. Try to rebound from one jump right into the next.

Trainer Tip: When performing a squat or a deadlift, concentrate on your posture. Keep your chest puffed up and pull your shoulder blades together. Be careful not to use your back too much. Most of your range of motion should come from your hips. And remember—butt out!

4. LUNGING

Lunges are one of the best exercises for toning and strengthening your legs and butt, two of the main areas that seem to concern my female clients, but don't think this lets you guys off the hook. Lunges should be a staple in everyone's fitness regimen. Just because you're not as worried about your butt, doesn't mean that lunges won't do you any good.

Lunges hit all the major parts of your lower body, get your heart pumping and will get the sweat pouring. Lunges are also great for revving up your metabolism because you are using so many large muscle groups at once (which is more or less the case for all of my top five). To perform a traditional lunge, stand upright and take a big step forward. Then lower yourself down until your back knee is just above the ground. Make sure to break the movement up into two phases: first forward and then down. A common mistake is taking the forward momentum into the downward phase, which might throw you off balance and lead to poor form. To work your legs evenly, you can alternate with each step, continuing forward in what is called a "walking lunge." They can also be done by stepping backwards (back lunge), side ways (you guessed it—side lunge), or any other way you can think to do them. There's even a stationary lunge called a "split squat."

Just like the squat, make sure you're getting a full range of motion out of each lunge. At the lowest point, your front knee should be bent at a 90-degree angle, making the top of your thigh parallel to the ground. Also, make sure to take a deep stride; you want to have at least a yard in between your front and back foot. For added resistance, you can perform lunges while holding dumbbells, resting a barbell on your back, using a kettlebell or any other way that you see fit. Get creative!

Trainer Tip: *Lunges*—When lunging, keep your front foot totally flat. Although the heel of your back foot ought to be up, don't let the heel of your front foot come up. Also, try to keep your back straight and don't allow your front knee to cross in front of your toes. Being mindful of these details will help you get the most out of each lunge.

5. STEPPING

Is your gym full of guys who want to show off their upper-body muscles while ignoring the rest of their bodies? Don't fall into this trap—there's more to strength training than bench presses and curls! In order to be truly fit, your entire body must be fit and able to function as a complete unit. Step-ups can help train your body to do just that. Take a break from the curls, step away from the mirror for a minute and get to work on the rest of your body.

When I suggest step-ups to people, they often ask, "What's the difference between this and just going up some stairs?" There's a BIG difference. Running stairs can be a great cardio workout, but it's not going to make your legs a whole lot stronger. When you do a step-up, you need your step to be higher than the stairs on a staircase. Doing a step-up onto a 6 inch step is like doing a squat and only going down 6-inches—it's not going to do much other than announce to anyone watching that you're a newbie. In order to really effect change in your muscles, use a step that puts your knee at a 90-degree angle when you plant your foot down.

To perform a basic step-up, first find something to step up on. Ideally, a flat surface at about knee height (a bench usually works well). Step up onto it and then lower yourself back down. Repeat the process with the other leg. Pretty simple, right? Bet you won't say that after doing twenty on each leg.

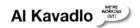
Once you get the movement down, you should start adding resistance to your step-ups by holding weights in your hands or resting a barbell across your back. You can perform step-ups by alternating legs or repeating the same leg for a set and then switching legs. I've found that in the context of conditioning workouts, alternating can sometimes be beneficial, whereas going one leg at a time is generally better for building strength.

Step-ups can also be performed laterally, by stepping onto a platform from the side. You can use a slightly lower step for this variation. Lateral step-ups work your inner thighs and hips, as well as your glutes, hamstrings and quads. Once again, what you do is up to you!

Trainer Tip: *Step-ups*—When performing a step-up, try to think about pushing through the heel of your foot as opposed to having all the weight on your toes. Also, be mindful of engaging your abdominal muscles on the way up in order to stay stable, this will improve the efficiency and effectiveness of each rep. Don't be afraid to test your limits with how much weight you can use on these. I've seen petite women perform step-ups for reps with barbells equal to half their body weight! They are not going to make your legs huge—just firm and toned!

6. DON'T FORGET TO STRETCH

Six? I thought you said only five! Yup, I did, but I had to sneak stretching in there because it's an important part of keeping your body healthy and ready for exercise. Also, I like to stretch after working out, so it seems fitting to discuss this here.

It's fairly common knowledge that flexibility is an important part of overall fitness. Most of us heard about it in gym class or from our high school coaches. Stretching can be a great way to cool down after a workout and it can reduce the likelihood of injury. Despite these well-known bonuses, lots of people leave stretching out of their regimen. Don't make this mistake.

Yes, I get it. I know why people don't like to stretch, it's boring. When you're all amped up from a workout sometimes you just don't feel like sitting down and stretching. I occasionally feel this way, too. Are there ways to avoid the boredom? Of course! Grab a friend!

Having a friend or trainer assist you can make stretching much more interesting and, in some cases, more effective. For example, if you want to stretch your hamstrings and inner thighs, start by sitting upright with your legs stretched out in front of you in a V shape. Have a partner sit across from you in the same position with their feet pressed up against yours. Then grab your partner's wrists and have them pull you in. Keep your back straight and your chest up. Take the stretch in your hips and legs. Hold the stretch for at least twenty seconds and then switch positions to help your partner stretch.

If you want to stretch your chest and shoulders, sit with your hands behind your head, fingers laced together and elbows out. Have your partner stand behind you and pull back on your elbows. It may be helpful to have your partner's knee or torso pressed against your back for leverage, but be careful with this. It's important to be verbal with your partner, so they don't overstretch you. Hold the stretch for at least twenty seconds.

As you are stretching, remember to keep your calm. Of course, thinking about relaxing sometimes makes it harder to do, so if you find yourself unable to focus, simply go back to your breathing. Concentrate on each breath as it goes fully in and fully out. This will help you relax and enhance your stretch. Physiologically, deep breathing gives your body the signal to calm down, which will facilitate a deeper stretch. Remember when we did that breathing exercise? This is yet another example of how your breath is tied to every aspect of your workout. Pay attention to your breath and you'll improve your workout and your stretching.

These two stretching examples I gave are just that: examples. There are hundreds of different ways to stretch. Stretching doesn't have to be boring, if you make it a part of your routine, you'll start to like it. Yoga has become increasingly popular and is a fun way to improve your flexibility (and strength!). Most forms of yoga center on the union of the mind and body. Like practicing mindfulness, practicing yoga can help increase focus and have a peaceful effect.

Yoga is one of those things that is best learned from an instructor, but like with any teacher, make sure you agree with what he or she is doing. Don't blindly listen to

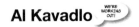

an instructor just because they're supposed to know more than you. There are a slew of yoga styles to choose from and some of them are really intense. This is fine as long as you're comfortable with it, but if the instructor is so extreme that you're doing things you don't want to do or pushing yourself beyond where you feel you should, don't be afraid to stop and find someone else. No one knows your body as well as you do, no matter what they say, so listen to what it's telling you.

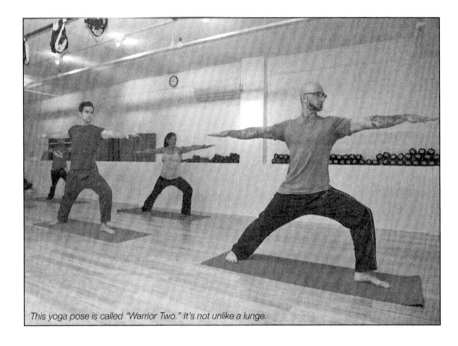
This yoga pose is called "Warrior Two." It's not unlike a lunge.

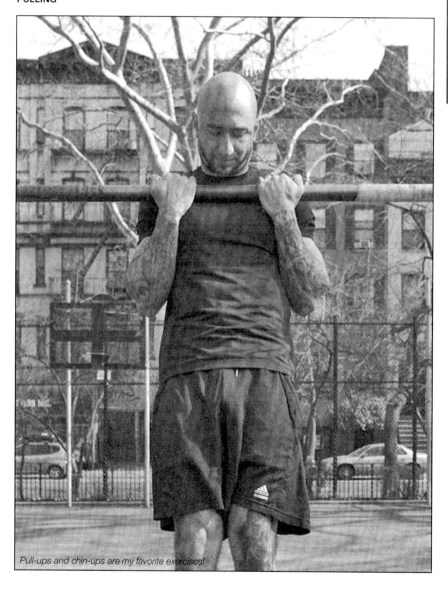

Pull-ups and chin-ups are my favorite exercises!

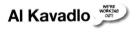

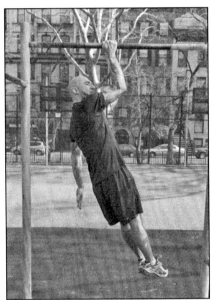
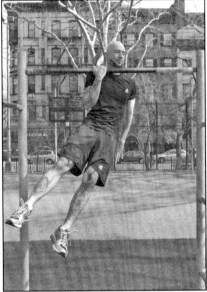
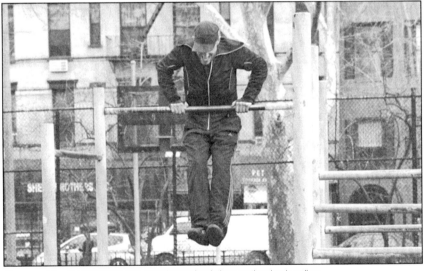

One arm chin-ups and muscle-ups are advanced variations on the classic pull-up.

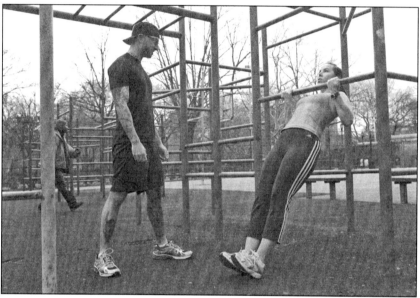

Australian pull-ups and rows are similar movement patterns.

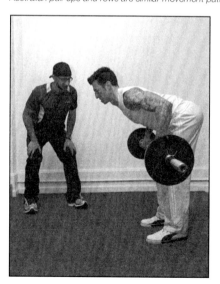

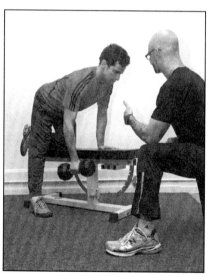

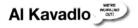
PUSHING

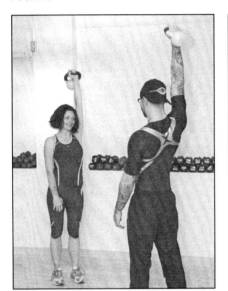
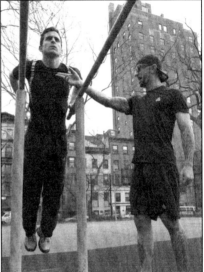
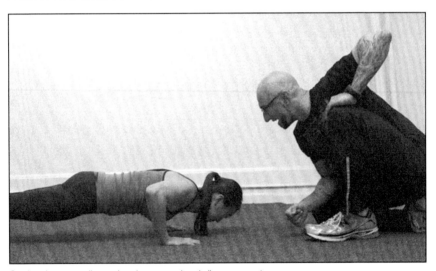

Overhead presses, dips and push-ups are also similar movements.

SQUATTING

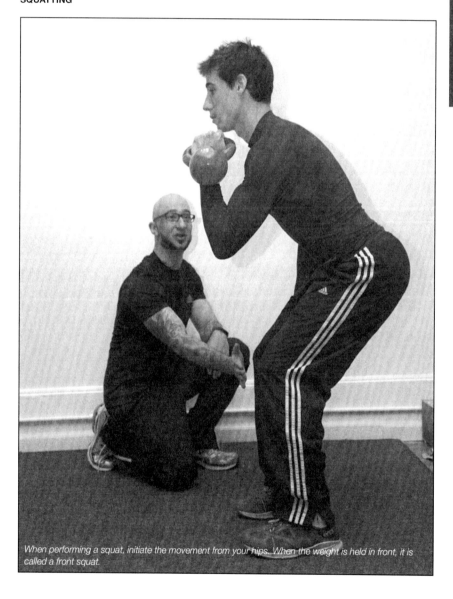

When performing a squat, initiate the movement from your hips. When the weight is held in front, it is called a front squat.

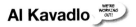

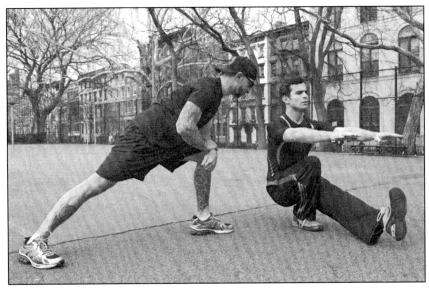

Whether you're performing a one-legged pistol squat or a traditional barbell back squat, stay mindful of keeping your back straight.

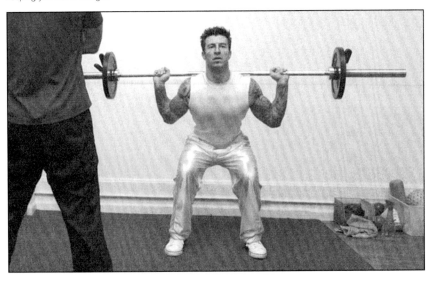

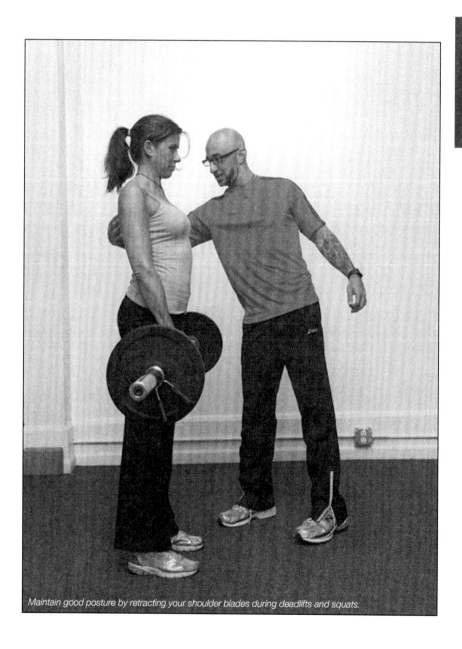

Maintain good posture by retracting your shoulder blades during deadlifts and squats.

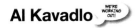
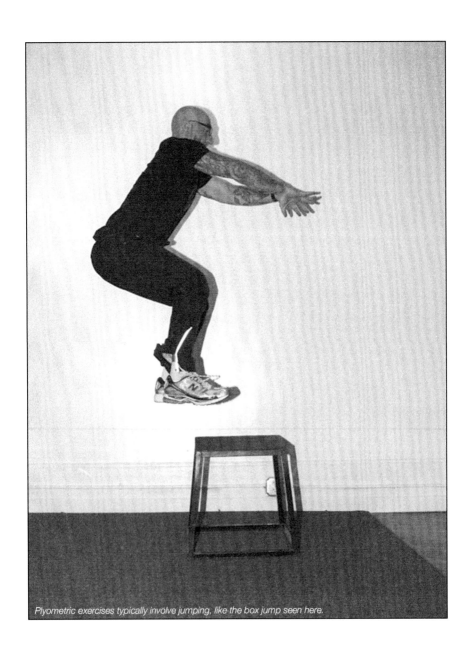

Plyometric exercises typically involve jumping, like the box jump seen here.

LUNGING

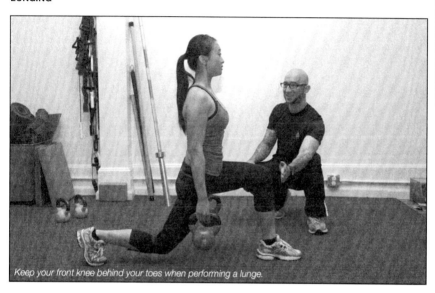

Keep your front knee behind your toes when performing a lunge.

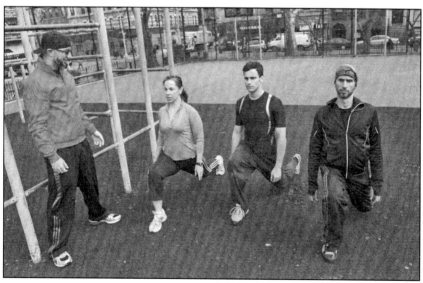

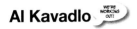

STEPPING

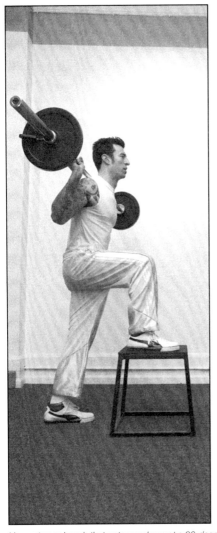 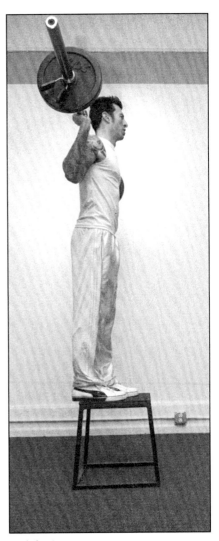

Use a step or bench that puts your knee at a 90-degree angle for step-ups.

STRETCHING

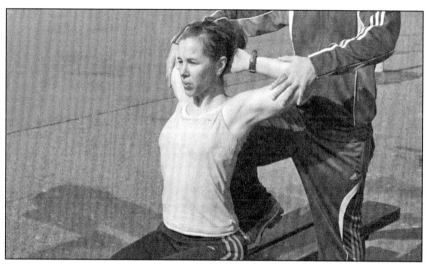

Stretching can be more fun with a buddy!

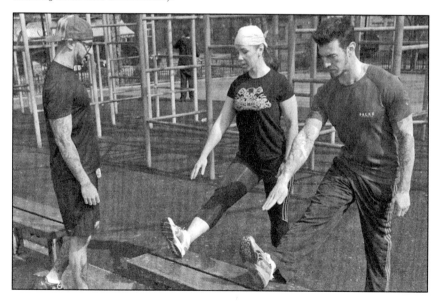

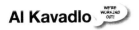

Chapter Six:
Primitive Minds: Fight or Flight

There are two basic responses when a person is presented with a threatening situation: you either run or you fight. This "fight or flight" response is something most of us learned about in high school health class. When in danger, your body floods itself with adrenaline, giving you the extra energy and strength you need to survive the situation. You decide to either stand your ground or cut and run.

While our ancestors were thrust into serious fight or flight situations on a regular basis, the average American doesn't come across these scenarios all that often. Neanderthal man was kept on edge by his constant contact with wild animals and warring neighbors. In comparison, we have it pretty easy. Yes, there are still things to keep us on guard; violent crimes happen every day (especially in NYC where I live). As a society, however, we've managed to remove most of the dangerous and threatening scenarios that plagued our ancestors. There are no roving wolf packs looking to steal our children or rivals trying to steal our resources. It's easy for us to relax and become complacent, but complacency is not our natural state.

With the lack of existing fight or flight scenarios, people have felt the urge to invent them. There is a primal need that must be sated, and that's where modern day running and martial arts come into play. With this in mind, a couple years ago I decided to try them both. After all, these two reactions are the most basic and natural forms of exercise.

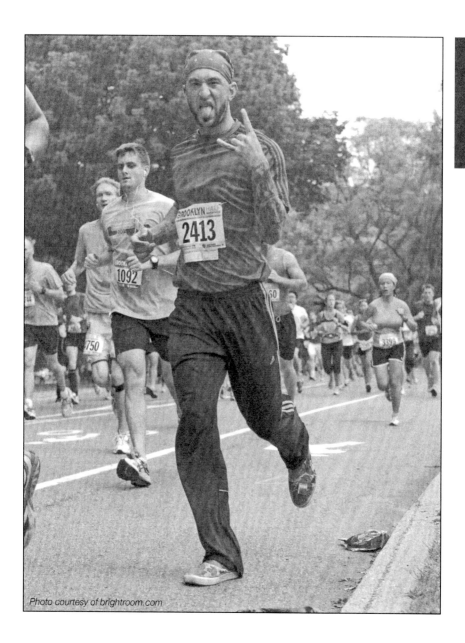

Photo courtesy of brightroom.com

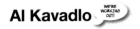

Al Kavadlo

RUNNING

As running was essential to the survival of primitive man, our bodies developed in a way that allows us to run for absurdly long distances with little wear. There are few other animals that are capable of comparable long distance running, and I don't think any of them do it for fun. We humans were born to run and it's an urge that many can't fight, including me. While my early experience with running was just as a means to get a six-pack, I eventually began to enjoy the process. Though I didn't learn to appreciate running until adulthood, I've been happily doing it for several years now.

I think every recreational runner should participate in an official race at some point. It will not only give you motivation and accountability, but come race day, the anxiety and anticipation you're bound to feel will be closer to a real a fight or flight situation. My first race was a 5K (3.1 miles) and I only participated in it as a favor to a co-worker. It was her first race, too, and she didn't want to do it alone. After weeks of nagging, I begrudgingly agreed to run with her. Initially, 5K seemed like an absurdly long distance to me. What was I getting myself into? How could I keep up my speed for that long? Could I finish without having to walk?

I still remember what it feels like to barely be able to run a mile. That was how I started, though, by conditioning myself to just run one mile. Gradually I was able to build upon that foundation. With time and practice, the 5K was soon behind me and I was sprinting towards a 10K. The 10K gave way to the half marathon, and the half marathon to the full. I ran my first marathon last year in New York City. It was an overwhelming and amazing experience.

The race itself was incredible. The excitement of the crowds, the support of friends and family and the beauty of New York City all served to make for an unforgettable day. The highs were some of the most amazing moments of my life and the lows were among the hardest. I felt great for most of the first three hours of the race, but around mile nineteen or twenty, my legs started to really feel fatigued. My original plan was to finish in under four hours, but I knew I couldn't keep up a nine-minute-mile pace much longer and if I tried I would be asking for trouble. As I've said, it's always important to listen to your body. Pushing yourself is good, but not at the risk of injury. At that point the game plan simply became to finish the race. From then on I decided that even if I had to slow down, hell, even if I had to crawl, I was not going to stop until I crossed the finish line.

When you run a marathon, you go through just about every emotion out there. As you're running, it's simultaneously the best thing you've ever done and the worst. It's important to be there for both extremes, though. You shouldn't try to block everything out when things get bad; you should pay attention to what you're doing and be there for every grueling moment. It builds character. Also, because I was present and concentrating on each stride I took, I knew that I needed to back off a little in order to keep on going. Whenever my mind began to wander, I would bring it back to the task at hand.

I finally finished at 4:22:11, which averages out to exactly a ten-minute-mile pace. The feeling of crossing the finish line is a hard thing to try to put into words. It was an exhilarating feeling and the culmination of years of hard work, but it was soon followed by one of the worst feelings in the world. When you finish a marathon it hurts to walk. The only thing that hurts more than walking is having to stop and stand, and that's exactly what you have to do for a good twenty or thirty minutes afterward. While everyone is huddled together trying to get their bags, take photos and meet with loved ones, there is nothing to do but stand there with your quads quivering and wait (another good exercise in patience and mindfulness). In spite of the struggle over the last several miles and the post-race discomfort, the marathon was an absolute blast! I plan on doing another marathon at some point, but my next several races have been shorter distances.

Running has become one of my favorite activities. It fulfills that ancient longing and it is one of the most effective forms of exercise out there. I don't want to go too deeply into running styles (that's a whole other book!), but as a general rule, try not to work too hard. Didn't expect me to say that, did you? It's true, though. Instead of trying to propel yourself off the ground, try to work with gravity and momentum. Don't go up, go forward. With each stride, lean forward and let the earth propel you and your foot. When you make contact, shift your weight and lean forward on the other leg. It's all about the transference of energy. Think of it as a continuous,

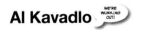

controlled fall. By letting gravity do the work, you're not only conserving energy, you're also running in a less stressful manner. Try to be light on your feet and stay off your heels to reduce impact—your knees and ankles will thank you.

MARTIAL ARTS

Fighting is as natural for us as running. Within each of us is a primitive beast that will lash out when in danger. It is our last resort and our last line of defense. Like running, however, fighting is not essential in our normal, everyday lives. Aside from a few small skirmishes, most people have never even been in a fight. Now don't get me wrong here, there's nothing at all wrong with that! I'm not advocating violence or encouraging people to fight unnecessarily (I'm a pacifist, man). I'm simply pointing out that there is that ability within all of us and it's not something that has to be ignored or frowned upon. In a controlled setting, martial arts can be a great way to exercise, get some aggression out and further learn to understand your body. There are many disciplines to choose from—some center on kicking, some on punching and some on grappling. There are many different options, but each will work your entire body and help strengthen the mind/body connection. And as an added bonus, if someone messes with you, you'll know how to handle yourself.

I studied Tae Kwon Do (a martial art centered around kicks and punches) for about six months when I was kid. It was one of those classes where you stand in lines with about fifteen other kids and yell "Hy-ah!" with every punch combination. My teacher wasn't exactly Mr. Myagi (we'll get to him in a minute), but it was a good class and I learned a lot. In addition to being a constructive way to get out all that extra kid energy, it taught me some discipline (and how to kick a little ass). One thing that stuck with me was something my teacher said to me about punching. He saw me punching a bag and came to observe more closely. After watching for a couple seconds, he stopped me and said, "Don't punch the bag, punch through it." This was a little confusing to me at the time, but I've thought about it since and I now have a better understanding. He didn't want me to explode the bag, he just meant that I should punch past the impact point. The reason for this is simple, if you're punching something (or someone) and you aim for the point at which impact will be made, then your punch will have no power. You need to aim beyond the point you can see, towards something deeper. This is great advice for fighting or fitness, but it's also a lesson that can be applied to life in general. If you planned to work out for a half hour and you're approaching the final couple of minutes, try shooting for an extra five minutes. Aim past your original goal. If you can't make it, that's fine. Sometimes it's good to have a goal that you can't reach. Remember, it's about right now; goals are just a fantasy.

When I hit high school, I took a break from martial arts and decided to bulk up instead. I was a skinny kid in a rough neighborhood and I wanted to put on a little muscle. I've continued strength training to this day, but a couple years ago, I decided to get back into fighting. I'm always on the lookout for new ways to exercise and I wanted to see how the Zen aspect could be applied to a different form of body manipulation. The more varied your workout, the less likely it is to get stale. MMA (mixed martial arts) and Brazilian Jiu-jitsu had just started to break into the mainstream, so I thought I'd give Jiu-jitsu a try.

Brazilian Jiu-jitsu is a grappling based martial art that started in Japan and made its way to Brazil, and more recently, to the United States. It is centered on submissions and pins, as opposed to punches and kicks. The general idea is through proper technique and the use of leverage, you use an attacker's energy against him instead of opposing it directly. This fighting style allows a smaller fighter to defeat a larger, and potentially stronger, opponent.

What interested me about Brazilian Jiu-jitsu is the manipulation of leverage and the transferring of energy. Just imagine the concentration and timing necessary to disarm and defeat an opponent with only your hands. Your opponent may seem to have the advantage, but if you are confident in your mind and body, you have complete control over your energy and even theirs. This is the type of concentration that you should take into every workout—exercise like your life depends on it, because in many ways, it does. Know how each muscle moves and how each rep or stride should feel. Harness your energy and adjust as you go along. Move with it and maximize each session. If you can maintain this type of focus, you can improve your workout tremendously.

I studied Brazilian Jiu-jitsu for just over a year before deciding that it wasn't for me (not very long, I know). I enjoyed certain aspects of it and learned a lot about

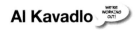

my body and myself. I gave it my all and I feel good about trying it. I worked on muscles that I'd rarely used elsewhere and learned more about leverage and energy transfers. It was definitely a cool and rewarding experience, but there's a downside to fighting. When you're fighting all the time, it's hard to keep from getting injured. The more fights you're in, the more you get hurt. This is just a part of fighting—I understand that. However, the injuries started interfering with other aspects of my life. When you're out every once in a while with a twisted knee or a tweaked back, it's hard to maintain a consistent running regimen, and running wasn't something I was willing to give up. I am glad I spent the time studying Brazilian Jiu-jitsu. New experiences are always worth the effort and often yield surprising results, whether that means increasing balance and awareness or disabling an armed attacker.

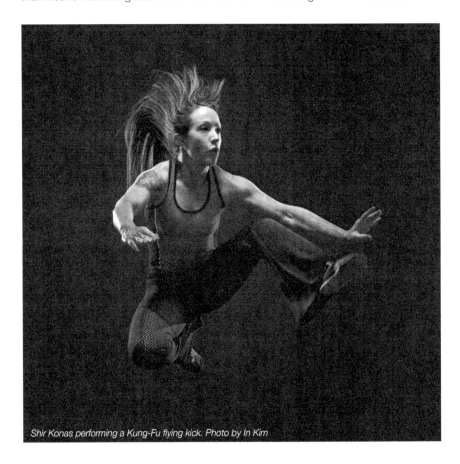

Shir Konas performing a Kung-Fu flying kick. Photo by In Kim

As I said earlier, studying a martial art is a great way to help you achieve harmony between your body and your mind. The longer you study a martial art, the more you will realize how much your body is capable of doing. The only thing holding you back is your mind. Over time, as you are able to free yourself from doubt and join your mind and body together, the limitations will appear to recede and you'll come to realize your greater potential. Of course, like Zen mindfulness and fitness, this takes time and hard work. Practice is the key.

THE MIND/BODY CONNECTION

When discussing the mind/body connection, I can't help but bring up *The Karate Kid*. If you're trying to wrap your head around the merits of hard work and practice and how they relate to the mind and body, look no further than Daniel and the teachings of Mr. Myagi.

After seeing Daniel get picked on and beaten up by the local thugs, Mr. Myagi agrees to train him in Karate. Naturally, Daniel is all excited about learning how to kick some ass, but when he shows up on the first day, what does Mr. Myagi tell him to do? Go wax those twenty cars (wax on, wax off). And the next day? Go paint that fence (up and down). And the next day? Go paint the house (left and right). Daniel begrudgingly sets about these tasks, but fails to see the point. Of course, he finally snaps at Mr. Myagi, demanding to know why he has to complete all these meaningless tasks. Unfazed by Daniel's outburst, Myagi tells Daniel to ready himself and begins throwing punches. With each punch, he yells out a command, "Paint the fence!" "Wax on!" "Wax off!" Daniel blocks each punch without difficulty, using each chore's motion to block the punches. Without realizing it, he has learned the basics of Karate and has built a foundation to learn more. He has learned discipline and mindfulness! Of course, it's not that quick or easy in real life, but hey, that's Hollywood for you.

As a quick aside here, I'd like to point out something else about Mr. Myagi. He's the epitome of functional strength. When confronted, he's able to take out Daniel's four attackers not because he has bulging biceps or ripped pecs, but because of his ability to harness energy and power from his core, utilizing his full strength. I know this is just a movie and that it's a little ridiculous to analyze it too deeply, but you can still learn a lesson from it.

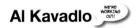

Al Kavadlo

Whether you're in a fight for your life or simply running at the track, concentrate, focus and utilize your entire body. The important thing is to commit yourself to the process. The more you give to the workout, the more it will give to you.

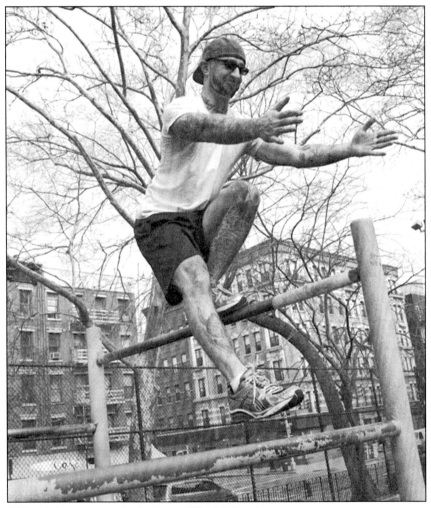

Adding a balance component makes for an additional challenge!

Chapter Seven:
Aesthetics vs. Functionality

Fitness, like many things, moves in trends. When I was growing up, for example, big muscles were in. People didn't just want to be fit, they wanted to be jacked. If you didn't have abs like Stallone and biceps like Schwarzenegger, you didn't have anything. The motto was, "The bigger, the better." This type of trend is great in terms of motivating people to push each other to higher levels of fitness, but it had dangerous and sometimes tragic repercussions as well. Athletes, pressured by society's obsession with size and Herculean strength, were pushing the envelope. Unfortunately, this led to the abuse of steroids and other performance enhancing drugs, which continues to be an issue with athletes of all kinds.

As a kid, I idolized wrestlers. There was Hulk Hogan, The Ultimate Warrior, and of course, Jesse "The Body" Ventura. They were AWESOME. Dressed in various colors of spandex, these beasts would come out to the ring, cheered on by ecstatic crowds and just annihilate each other. They looked like titans or mythic gods. That's what I aspired toward; that was my first glimpse into the world of fitness. And it was pure vanity. People only cared about how they looked and not how they felt.

Still, I wanted to look like these guys! I put them on a pedestal but, as it turns out, that's not really what I wanted at all. These men weren't the epitome of health, virility or fitness. They overstressed and overtaxed their bodies and now many of them are paying for it with back pain, joint trouble or worse. Their physiques were unnatural and unhealthy and their bodies eventually paid the price. There is a lesson to learn

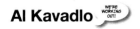

Al Kavadlo

from this: don't overdo it. Don't get lost in a quest for image. Keep your head about you and pay attention to what you're doing and how your body is reacting. Big muscles are worthless if your joints are too weak to use them.

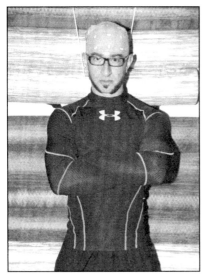

Fortunately, the vibe in fitness is changing. We're trending towards health and functionality, instead of aesthetics. The bulky, bodybuilder look is slowly fading out of favor. Instead of being the next Arnold, people simply want to be fit and lean. Thankfully, the idea that fitness is just about looking good is starting to become outdated. Now, don't get me wrong here, I have great respect for bodybuilders. They are able to accomplish amazing things, but bodybuilding is about aesthetics, achieving a particular look, not about practicality. Now the focus is on feeling good and being healthy. Basically, it's a change of priorities. Many people are now focusing first on functionality, on what they can do with their bodies, and not worrying as much about appearance. Looks are no longer the emphasis, but more like an added bonus.

What do I mean by functionality? Let me use bodybuilders as an example. Last year, over 40,000 people ran the New York City Marathon. If you took a bodybuilder and threw him into the race, he probably wouldn't make it past the first few miles. If you threw him into the ring (or cage) with a Jiu-jitsu fighter, he'd probably get his ass handed to him. Sure, he's got more muscle than both the runner and the martial artist, but he can't effectively utilize it in these scenarios. His muscles are for show, while the other athlete's overall fitness is for functionality. They are more versatile and able to make use of their respective strengths. The bodybuilder is a bit more limited. It's simply a matter of goals. Bodybuilders want to impress the judges, while the modern exerciser wants to become fit in order to do more, whether that means hiking with friends, running a marathon or just chasing after your kids. At the marathon, I saw a 75-year-old blind woman running the race. And you know what? She finished! It took her eight hours but she crossed that finish line. Now, tell me that's not badass? This is the type of attitude I'm talking about, exercising in order to keep moving and keep active; exercising in order to not be held back.

This is an exciting time to start getting fit, so don't make any more excuses!

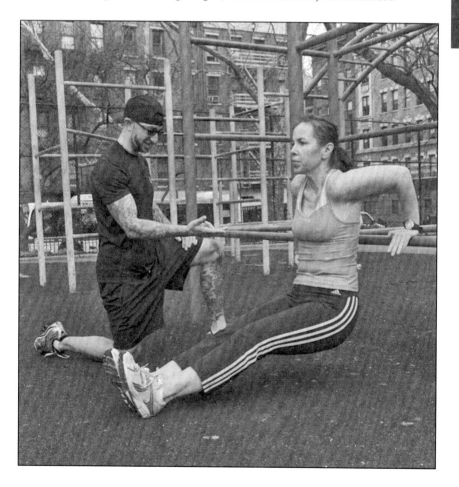

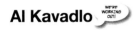
Chapter Eight:
Fifty-Fifty

The way I look at it, life is pretty much fifty-fifty. On its own, no individual thing is entirely good or entirely bad. There are pros and cons to all situations.

People always ask me to tell them the best way to get fit. Like I told you, everything has its pros and cons, there is no best way—just stay consistently active and mindful. Once you do that, you'll see for yourself what works and what doesn't. You can go to a gym or you can stay in your house; you can work out alone or with a friend; you can hire a trainer or you can experiment for yourself. ALL of these are good options, but since people insist on asking me which I think are the best, we'll go through the pros and cons of each. Fifty-fifty.

THE GYM

Pros: The gym can be a great place to work out. It has just about everything you could possibly need to get fit, but more importantly, it's a destination. It's a place that requires you to leave the comfort of your home and the habits associated with it. Once you've made it to the gym, there's not much to do but exercise. It's much easier to pick up a dumbbell when there's a roomful of people already working out. The further away from your couch you are, the more likely you are to exercise. In addition, a fully stocked gym allows you to vary your workout easily, which keeps your regimen fresh and exciting, at least in theory. Working out at home can seem a little repetitive, and without more equipment on hand, it can be tough to change things up. If you're at the gym, you can switch from leg presses to bench presses with ease. All in all, gyms have options, like equipment, classes and trainers, which can help keep you on track. Oddly enough, most people at the gym seem to do the same two or three things every time anyway.

Cons: Some people just don't like the gym. Instead of being an encouraging environment, it can be an intimidating place. In addition, gyms can be expensive. If you don't have disposable income, a gym membership may be out of your reach. While there is a lot of equipment in the gym, all of it isn't totally necessary. You can get fit with no equipment at all, using only your body. As long as you're committed to getting fit, there are endless ways to exercise and make a positive change. Go to the park, go for a jog or a hike, meet some friends for a game of basketball—it doesn't matter where you do something, as long as you're doing it.

I need to address these cons a bit more, I can't help myself. In terms of the intimidating aspect of some gyms, the key is to not let this get to you. Everything is a little intimidating at first, but the more you do it, the more comfortable you get. In short, suck it up. It's not that bad. If you don't know where to start, don't get overwhelmed. Look at the gym like a shoe store; when you're in there, surrounded by shoes, it can be tough to pick out which ones you like. So what do you do? Get embarrassed, hang your head and run out? No, you suck it up and start trying on shoes; when you're at the gym, do the same thing. Just pick something and give it a whirl. If it's a good fit, try it again next time. If it's not, try something else. Also, keep in mind that everyone is there for the same reason—exercise. As for the cost of a gym membership, yes, it can get expensive. Some people can't afford it and that's fine. Don't let this stop you from working out in your house or somewhere outside. There are plenty of free places, so don't use money as an excuse to sit on your ass! My favorite place to work out is Tompkins Square Park—my neighborhood park in NYC. It's free and I don't even have to leave the East Village. There are no pretentious people and everyone who shows up is there to work hard and have fun. If you're hesitant about the gym, check out some parks in your area.

The answer to your question is: it doesn't matter! Gym or no gym, it's all up to you! No one can do this for you, so just pick something and stick to it. If you get bored, try something else. Just keep moving.

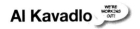
WORKOUT BUDDIES

Pros: Working out with a friend is a great way to stay motivated. If you can start thinking of the gym as a place where you can not only work out, but a place where you can spend time with your buddy, it can make a big difference in the way you approach exercise. This comes back to the idea of enjoying your workout experience. If you like going, you're more likely to keep going and keep improving.

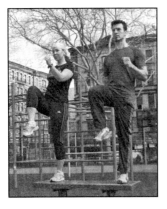

A friend can also be helpful once you're in the gym. Most people are naturally competitive; no one likes to be the one holding the group back. As a result, people working out in pairs often push one another and work harder than they would if they were alone. Hopefully, our competitive streaks will keep us from slacking off and doing the same old routine.

Cons: Working out with a friend can sometimes hold you back. First, you need to find a friend whose fitness level is similar to yours. If one of you is way ahead (or way behind), it makes it hard to motivate one another. It's no fun to start a run with your buddy and then have them drop you because you can't match their pace. Conversely, it's not as fun (nor as effective) to run with someone who is holding you back. There's also a risk of becoming too dependent on your friend's support. If you and your friend are in a yoga class together, but she moves away, your motivation might move right along with her.

Another caution: be careful your gym buddy doesn't turn into your bullshit buddy. Every day I see people standing around talking and laughing at the juice bar or by the bench presses. Now don't get me wrong, this is great. It's important to enjoy exercise and make the gym a fun place to be, but don't forget why you are there! Just being at the gym isn't what makes you fit—you have to work! Chatting and laughing is all well and good, but not if it's getting in the way of your workout. What am I saying? If you want to work out with a friend, be sure it's one that takes fitness seriously.

What's the answer to this one? Simple, if you have a friend you'd like to work out with, then do it. Just don't get so wrapped up that you can't enjoy exercising when they're not around. If you don't have a friend at the same level, no big deal; exercise can still be enjoyed on its own. You don't need someone else next to you while you're doing push-ups, you can handle it. Don't be afraid to be alone. That said, if you find yourself getting bored or complacent, try joining a class or working with a trainer.

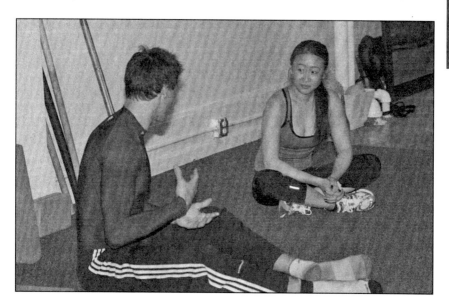

HIRING A TRAINER

Pros: As a personal trainer myself, this is a pretty easy one to answer. Yes, if you're serious about getting fit, you should hire a personal trainer. They give you the same benefits as working out with a friend (motivation, competition, energy, etc.), and few of the possible negatives (laziness, different fitness levels, bullshit buddy, etc.). A good trainer has the knowledge and the know-how to help you take your workout to the next level. You don't have to worry about what they're doing or what their fitness level is because it doesn't matter; they are there for you. Their goal is to get

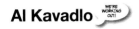

you fit. Don't forget that trainers are people, too, though! (Once you get to know them, trainers can become bullshit buddies, too. Be sure to keep your trainer on track, just like they should keep you on track.)

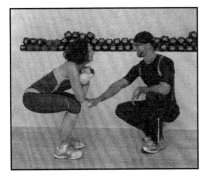

Having a trainer can help provide the necessary motivation and structure to your routine that you need, but essentially it comes down to accountability. A lot of us can rationalize letting ourselves down, but when we have someone else that is relying on us or watching us, our sense of responsibility kicks in and we tend to step it up and get it done. When you have a trainer as that "someone," they can help motivate and push you, as well as educate you. Having a trainer direct your workout also frees up your mind. You can simply focus on the task at hand and practice paying attention to the workout, focusing on the present and not worrying about what comes next. Let the trainer worry about the next exercise, while you simply concentrate on the movement of your body.

Cons: The financial expense is really the only con to having a good trainer. Like gym memberships, personal trainers cost money. Are they a worthwhile investment? Yes, definitely. Everybody needs training and everybody has the potential to improve, so why wouldn't you want to have someone around who can help you with both? However, if you're short on money, it becomes a tough decision. If you can't afford it, you can't afford it. It's as simple as that. But if you're on the fence, think of it as a quality of life question. If you're overweight and it's affecting your life, whether that means you can't keep up with your kids, get a date or your health is in jeopardy, then this is something that could greatly improve your quality of life. For some, a trainer is a luxury, but for others, it's a necessity. If you need one, don't get caught up in the extra couple of dollars. Bite the bullet and get it done. Hiring a trainer can be the first step towards improving your health and fitness. However don't fall into the trap of thinking that just because you hire a trainer, you'll magically be fit. You still need to do the work!

When hiring a trainer, keep in mind that all trainers are not created equal. If you live in a small town, you might not have a plethora of choices. On the other hand, if you live in a big city, there are more options. When you pick a trainer, try to choose one that has some experience. Of course, as the quality of the trainer goes up, so does the amount they charge. If you can afford the best, good for you, get the best. For those of you who can't, you might be able to find somebody who is willing to work with you on the price if they know you're willing to commit to training with them for an extended period of time. Most trainers offer volume discounts, and big training packages also help to keep you on track. Once you've already paid, you're more likely to show up! Money is tough, but don't be cheap. Your best bet is to ask around; people who love their trainers will usually spread the word. I put a lot more stock in referrals and word of mouth than I do in fancy sounding credentials. If you don't know anyone, then go to the gym and talk to some trainers until you find someone who you click with and feel you can trust. Don't be nervous about approaching them, they'll be happy to chat you up—you're a potential customer!

As you can see, there are no definitive answers to these questions, but that's the way of the world. No workout regimen is the be-all-and-end-all of workouts. Things change in life and that's okay. It's good to explore all your options. Like the tattoo across my neck says, nothing lasts forever. The only constant in life is that you will always be you and now will always be now. That's all we've got, so do the most with it.

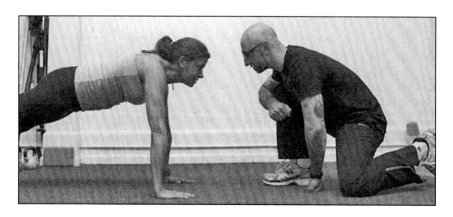

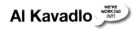

Chapter Nine:
The Level Playing Field and the Path Ahead

I come across a lot of people who somehow think that just by hiring me as their trainer, they will automatically become fit without having to work for it (but YOU know better than that by now, right?). Sometimes people get so used to being able to fix any problem just by throwing money at it that they expect getting fit to be the same. Well, it's not. It's unfortunate and kind of sad that some people have become accustomed to dealing with life in this manner. Using money instead of willpower is a detriment to motivation. Why try if you can just pay to get what you want?

Well, this question leads us to one of my favorite things about fitness: no matter who you are, how much money you have or who your cousin is, there are no shortcuts to getting in shape. You can hire the most expensive trainer in the world and you'll still have to put in the effort; the trainer can't do it for you. Even once you've achieved a high level of fitness, you can't just sit back and relax—if you stop working, it starts to go away. Exercise puts everyone on a level playing field—you can only get out of it as much as you're willing to put into it.

There are some misguided people at the gym who think just showing up is enough. Since they aren't making any real effort, they're not going to see much change. Eventually they'll start thinking it's hopeless, that they'll never get any fitter. They're going to the gym three or four times a week, how much more can they do?

You might have convinced yourself that exercise just doesn't work for you; however, the reality is that if you're not making progress, you probably aren't working for it. Just getting up on an elliptical trainer and lazily peddling away while you watch soap operas isn't much better than sitting on the couch and watching them. Don't get me wrong here, for a very deconditioned individual, a slow pace on an elliptical trainer might be a high enough intensity at first, but after a couple of weeks it will no longer be a challenge and the intensity will need to be increased. If you keep plodding along at the same slow pace, you're not going to improve. It doesn't matter how many days you show up at the gym if you're not going to push yourself while you are there.

As a general rule of thumb, if you aren't breaking a sweat, you need to increase your exercise intensity. The relative intensity of the workout is the key. A workout that might be hard for one person might be easy for another. A sedentary person might find riding a bicycle for thirty minutes at a ten mile-an-hour pace to be quite a challenge, but for someone like Lance Armstrong, it is barely a warm up. Of course, the average person shouldn't be comparing himself to elite athletes; my point is that you have to be realistic. You have to make sure that you're taking yourself to your limit. You fit folks should heed this warning as well. We've talked a little about the dangers of complacency; remember, if you don't keep striving forward, you'll plateau and then slowly start to slide back downhill. A good trainer can be a huge asset here. If they know what they are doing, they'll recognize the signs of this decline and cut it off at the pass.

Occasionally, clients of mine who aren't making progress will admit to me that they are not doing their part (although it's obvious who is and who isn't). Other times, people will go into denial and blame anyone and anything, but themselves. I have heard many excuses why people can't stick to a diet or exercise program, but they're all essentially the same: it's someone else's fault. They blame their boss, their family, heck, even the freakin' airport! Sometimes they say that as their trainer, it's my fault. People will often delude themselves into thinking there are things they simply can't overcome (time, money, etc.), so they won't have to put in the effort. It's ridiculous. You need to fight off that little weenie voice in your head that wants you to plop down on the couch with a pint of Hagen Daz. A trainer is like a tutor; they can provide you with information and knowledge, but they can't take the test for you, that part is up to you.

Al Kavadlo

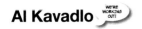

I'm reminded of a former client of mine (I'll call him Hank), who complained during every workout. I never really understood why he even bothered to show up, since he was rarely prepared to give any effort. I trained Hank for over a year and in that time he never achieved any significant weight loss or any increase in his performance. The couple of pounds that he would drop here and there would always come back on within the next few weeks. Their return somehow always coincided with Hank's business trips. Funny how that happened.

Throughout our time together, I would try different ways of dealing with Hank. In the beginning, I was very confident and optimistic, but over time, I became disillusioned. He would cancel appointments at the last minute or not give any serious effort when he actually showed up. Any time I pushed him to exert more than a minimal amount of effort it became an ordeal. He'd demand breaks even if he was only slightly out of breath or he'd whine that I was pushing him too hard. Occasionally, he'd come in with a different attitude and actually put in some real work, but it never lasted; the next week he'd cancel or come in with the same old excuses. The cycle repeated itself over and over until we'd eventually had enough of each other. The lesson here is that Hank never took responsibility for himself. He belonged to a gym and had a trainer, but he still couldn't get fit. If you asked him why, he'd probably say something like, "The program wasn't working for me." That was the problem—he was deluding himself into not taking responsibility. In order to be successful, in fitness or anything else, you need to grab the reins and make it happen. Hank wasn't only shying from the reins, he was jumping off the horse.

Even "good" clients of mine, those who work out hard and are usually pretty consistent, occasionally trick themselves into seeing things from a skewed perspective. The other day I received an e-mail from one of these clients (we'll call him Tony) that struck me as funny. He wrote:

"Hi, I haven't had any time to make it to the gym since our last session. Could we move tonight's session back to next week? If that doesn't work for you that is fine. Just thought I would get more out of it if I did some work on my own."

This type of "logic" is sadly quite prevalent. People think they need to somehow "get ready" for a workout. In actuality, the workout itself is the preparation. While consistent training is the only way to make any serious progress, putting off a workout because it's been a while since your last one is getting it backwards. Think about it—not working out because you haven't been working out? If you follow that logic, you'll never get anywhere.

The last sentence of the e-mail was the most interesting part. Tony displayed the "all or nothing" attitude that I mentioned earlier. He's right that he would get more out of training with me if he worked out more on his own, but by doing neither, he gets nothing. Something is always better than nothing. Even if it's just a twenty minute workout, it's better than no workout. You get it in when you can fit it in. I'm a reasonable person; I know you have other things in your life besides fitness. After all, what's the point of being well conditioned and fit if you can't enjoy it? (In case you were wondering, I convinced Tony to come in for the session and he had a great workout. He got through everything that I asked of him and he thanked me for not letting him dip out.)

All this "it's up to you" talk can be a bit much, I know. But if you look within yourself and decide to take full responsibility for where you are and how you got there, it can be really beneficial and not just in regard to fitness. Once you can accept and embrace that you are in control, you'll have a much better chance of being able to steer your body, and your life, in the direction you'd like. I know this might sound a little unrealistic. Getting fit isn't an easy thing to do and deciding to change your life and your habits is no small challenge either. The whole prospect can seem overwhelming, almost impossible, but it's not. It just takes time.

Have you ever been driving somewhere, missed an exit and didn't realize it until you'd already gone miles out the way? At some point, you know you've made a mistake and you have no choice but to go back the way you came. Even though you know there's really no other option, a part of your mind still doesn't want to accept the situation, doesn't want to turn around. You want to keep going the way you're headed and avoid the stress of the turn. This kind of irrational stubbornness is more common than we'd like to admit. You don't want to accept that you've been going down the wrong path for so long without even knowing it. You wish you could just keep going and somehow wind up at your destination, that turning

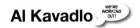
around isn't really necessary. But, in reality it doesn't work like that. Often, we will instinctively want to stay on the path we are on, even when it's clearly the wrong one, simply because it's comfortable. And when we are stuck on one path, the path of not exercising for example, that turn can seem like the hardest thing in the world.

Humans are habitual creatures; we get into patterns and get comfortable with them. The further you get down that unhealthy path, the more you will have to backtrack. Ironically, it is for precisely this reason that many people never begin an exercise program. They feel like they've gone so far down the path that there is no longer any hope for them. This is an unfortunate perspective to take, but that's all it is, a perspective. Remember, you are at the wheel, you're the one in charge. You can change your perspective; every day you have a choice, every moment of every

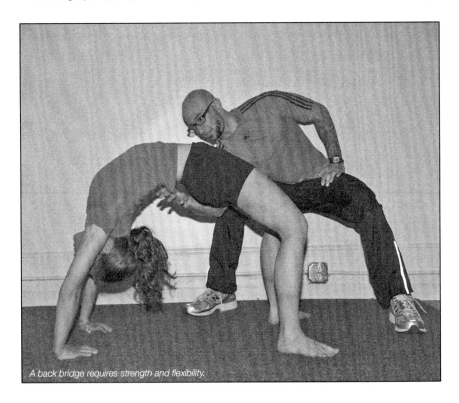

A back bridge requires strength and flexibility.

day, for that matter. Don't let your habits decide your destination, change them and shape them. You can go anywhere, you just need to make that first turn.

Every step you take down your new road will get a little easier. Not to say that there won't be a few bumpy parts here and there, but overall, it gets easier as you go along. Once you set good habits in place, just like the bad ones, they become a part of your thought patterns and the signals in your brain make them happen a little easier. That's right, I'm going to get into a quick neuroscience lesson now.

Our brains get our bodies to move by communicating with our muscles through an extremely complex system of nerve impulses. When a muscle gets the signal to move in a way that it's not used to (like doing a push-up if it has been a few months/years/decades/never), it takes a bit longer for the signal to get there and it may not get there clearly. So the movement, the push-up in this case, might not look very clean or feel very good. With repetition, the signal gets better at getting to the muscle. This is actually why people can appear to get a lot stronger quickly after they begin strength training. It's because they're not only building strength, they're also getting better at coordinating the movements. Over time and with consistent practice, exercises will eventually become second nature. Just like you don't need to give any thought to walking down the street or opening a door, an experienced weightlifter can perform a clean and jerk with little overt awareness of the mechanics of the lift. Improved body awareness is a wonderful benefit of exercise. The more aware you are of your body, the further you can push it while safely understanding its capabilities and limitations.

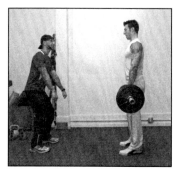

Imagine for a second that you wake up in a house in the middle of a thick rainforest, miles away from the closest town. You need supplies (food, water, etc.) and the only way to purchase them is to fight your way through the dense underbrush to get to town. So, you grab your machete and off you go. Your first trek to town is brutal; there's no path to follow, you're getting tripped up in the underbrush, your lungs are

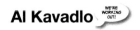

burning and your arm is aching from hacking your way through the trees. Finally, after what seems like an eternity, you reach town, exhausted and sore, but happy to have arrived.

The next trip to town will be a little less of a struggle. As you leave your house and start toward the edge of the woods, you can see where you went through the day before. Some branches are hacked and broken, and the ground is slightly trodden, but it still looks intimidating. You start to question whether you really need to go to town today (you were there yesterday, after all), but then you stop yourself; there's nothing to fear. You just did it the day before and you survived. So you take a deep breath, gather your thoughts, and off you go again, machete a swingin'. This time the trip is a little easier. The path is smoother, a little more forgiving. By focusing, you're able to find your footing and move swiftly along.

Now let's skip ahead to day twenty. With nineteen days under your belt, the path has been packed down and cleared so thoroughly that it's no longer a path, but a full-blown trail. Feeling fresh, you leave the machete behind and lope down your personalized trail. Now think back to that first grueling day and what it has turned into. The first is the worst (and it sucks), but that also means that every day after it will be better, easier.

I know I keep saying this, but despite what I've said above about "just doing it," deciding to get fit is not an easy thing to do. It takes time, willpower and confidence. But what I need to make you understand, is that it's possible for you (not me, or your friend, or an athlete, but YOU), to do it anyway. You simply need to believe that you can. Let's talk about this in terms of a pop culture reference again. Why? Because it's fun.

Right now, you're like Keanu Reeves in the beginning of *The Matrix* (fun, right?), when he swallows the red pill and wakes up in the "real world." When he comes to, bald, dressed in tattered clothing and on some sort of strange ship, his mind can't accept what's happening. He backs away from Morpheus and the rest of the crew, yelling at them to stay away from him and then vomits in the corner and passes out. In other words, he completely shuts down. He's been conditioned to believe that his old life in the matrix was real, but now he has to face the fact that it's not.

He has to go against everything his mind thought he knew. This is where you are. You're Keanu, collapsed in the corner, trying to fight your mind. You've conditioned yourself into thinking you can't get fit, that it's too hard. Like Keanu, you have a lot to learn.

As the movie progresses, Keanu learns to focus his mind and accept the possibility of success. He improves slightly, but is unable to reach his full potential. Why is that? Because, just like you, he doesn't yet believe that he can. And that's the whole trick. Like Keanu, YOU are The One. You have all the power and all the control. You simply need to believe in it and believe in yourself. Sounds a little cheesy, right? Well, tell that to Keanu. He saved the world.

HOW TO DO A HANDSTAND

(See photos on pages 88 and 89)

1. Reach your arms up.

2. Lean forward from your hips, keeping your back straight.

3. Kick up with one leg, shifting your weight into your hands.

4. Follow with your other leg, allowing your back to arch slightly.

5. Center your hips over your shoulders.

Practice against a wall to start out. Over time, as your balance improves, you can try to come away from the wall.

Trainer Tip: Look in between your hands and keep your arms straight as you kick up. Press your fingertips into the ground to prevent yourself from falling forward.

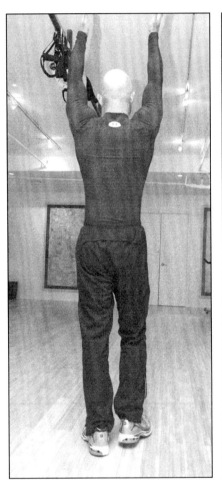 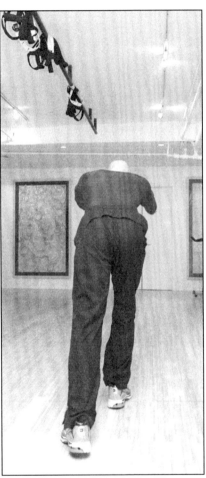

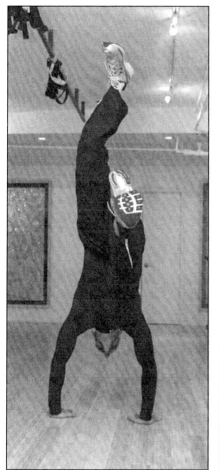
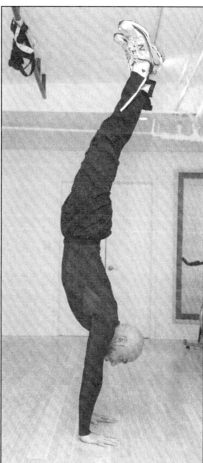

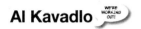

Chapter Ten:
We're Working Out!

At the beginning of this book I told you I wasn't going to bullshit you and I'm not going to do it here either. Getting fit isn't easy, no matter what any commercial or fitness "expert" tells you. However, I hope you've seen that it doesn't have to be a miserable experience. You can get fit and it can be fun! Before you walk away from this book (and go work out!), I want you to think about three things: your mindset, your body and your quality of life. They're all connected, like links in a chain. It starts with your mindset and from there you can create the body you want and the quality of life you deserve.

1. YOUR MINDSET

Achieving your fitness goals is a matter of willpower. You are as capable as anyone else; you just need to commit to the idea that change is possible and that you are going to do it. From there, you simply need to start. As you know, there will be times when it's hard, when the road is bumpier than you'd hoped. Life will constantly test and humble you. The key is to accept this and then deal with it day to day. You don't need to push yourself beyond your limits every single day. If you're feeling tired and sluggish one day, ease off a bit and do a less intense workout. The next day, you'll be pumped and ready to push the envelope. Listen to what your body is telling you each day and act accordingly. The important thing is to just keep getting out there. Remember on the days when you don't feel like it, willing yourself to do some light exercise will almost always leave you feeling better.

Think of your body as a rock that for years has been left essentially untouched by the elements, remaining smooth and unsculpted. As the mountains have thawed and water (your workout) has begun to run over it, that rock (you) will begin to adapt. The strength of the water varies from day to day, changing with the weather. Yesterday it was slow but steady, today a stream pooled and then overflowed, sending a fast current careening down the mountain and over your rock. After two days, the rock seems unaffected, but in truth, its surface is changing. The transformation, though slow, has begun.

It's not too hard to see where I'm going with this metaphor—water over time will wear down the rock, sculpting it as it pleases. Like the rock, sculpting your body takes time. It won't happen right away; you need to flow consistently, like the water. But don't forget, the water flows a little differently each day.

If it's been raining, the current will be faster, more intense. But if it's a lazy, no cloud in the sky kind of day, the water will stream down more gently, still running over the rock, but not putting as much stress on it. It varies like your workouts—hard on some days, easier on others. The important thing to note is the effect on your body. If you worked out really hard yesterday, then had a rough day today and could only fit in a shorter session, that's okay. Think about the rock. Two months from now, you won't be able to tell the difference. A couple of relaxed workouts aren't going to stop the rock from changing. As long as you're consistent, as long as you keep pouring water, at whatever speed, over that rock, it will change.

2. YOUR BODY
If you take one thing away from this book, make it this: TAKE CARE OF YOUR BODY! If you wake up each day with this idea in your head, that's a good start. In order to improve your fitness level, you simply have to make better decisions. Treat your body with respect by exercising and eating a healthy diet.

I talked about diet in Chapter Two, so it might not be fresh in your mind. The most important thing to remember is that mess-ups happen. While you should strive to avoid junk food and processed garbage like McDonald's, there will be a day sometime in the future when you'll say, "Ah, what the hell. Let me get the double cheeseburger combo." It's going to happen, BUT IT'S NOT A BIG DEAL. So many people give up on themselves because of a slip-up. Instead of abandoning ship, just get back at the helm and start moving in the right direction. But remember, your

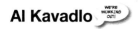
Al Kavadlo

choices add up. Playing the "next time" game too often can turn into the "all the time" game. Before you know it, you're back at square one. Your mindset is just the beginning; if you can't put that plan into action, then it's just a useless, flabby plan. You need to make it happen!

This principle applies to your workout schedule, too. Of course, you should take it day by day. If something urgent comes up (sickness, family obligations, etc.) and interrupts your program, don't freak out about it. While daily exercise is ideal, missing a day or even a week is not the end of the world. Sure, not working out for a while will set you back, but don't let that stop you from starting again. Remember our car example from a couple chapters back? Don't head in the wrong direction just because it's easier than turning around. The beauty of life is that each day brings with it a blank slate. It doesn't matter what you did the day before because that's in the past. It's a harsh reality of life—all that matters is what you've done lately—but it's also empowering. When you wake up, you have anything and everything ahead of you. If you didn't work out yesterday, that's fine, just be sure to get out there today. Live in the moment and remember that there's no better time to start than now.

You only get one body, but you have the opportunity to shape that body to your liking. Every day provides an infinite number of possibilities. It's simple, just take care of your body. It's the only one you're gonna get, so you might as well treat it right. Tired of being fat and weak? Do something about it! Get up, get out and get started.

3. QUALITY OF LIFE

Getting fit isn't about appearance; it's about your quality of life. Maybe you're not fat and you don't feel weak, but you can always improve yourself. You won't know until you try. Don't let your laziness keep you from living your life. As Buddha himself once said, "We are all the authors of our own health or disease." If you're seriously overweight, you're putting yourself at risk for a lot of health problems and chances are you already know this. Hopefully that's one of the reasons why you're reading this book. And that's good! You've taken the first step. Now take the next and the next and the next. Go for a run, play a game of tennis, start living your life and feeling good!

Living a healthy lifestyle doesn't have to be something you dread. Take a class, join a soccer team, practice yoga or start rock climbing. There are endless ways to get fit. You don't need to limit yourself. Get out there and find something you like, something that challenges and excites you. You can enjoy getting fit. As I told you in the beginning: starting is tough, but as you continue on and make exercise a part of your routine, it not only becomes easier, it becomes enjoyable. Give it time and you'll start to like it.

I GOTTA SAY IT AGAIN

Anyone who tells you that they have a secret about how to get in shape, lose weight or improve your life is probably full of shit. Sure, some of these things might give you a quick fix, but in the big picture, there are no short cuts. Even though we all know this deep down, it's still hard to let go of the fantasy that life will one day magically get easier. I catch myself doing it too sometimes. When you're thinking about long term fitness, you cannot be short-sighted. Everyone knows the story of the tortoise and the hare, but few take that lesson to heart. You need to work at it, keep moving, however slow the pace.

As I mentioned earlier, I went through a brief martial arts phase when I was a kid. I was young, so I honestly don't recall all that much about it, but I do remember why I stopped. I stopped because I was bad at it. One day my mom picked me up after class and I was exhausted and frustrated. I told her that I didn't think I wanted to do it anymore and she simply said, "Fine." It was that easy. I complained all the time about school, but I still had to keep going back there. Same with chores. It didn't matter how bad I was at washing dishes, I could never get out of doing them. For the first time, just being bad at something and not wanting to do it anymore was actually enough. Mom just said, "Fine." Of course, in retrospect, I see it more from my mom's point of view. I have a wonderful mother, I am very lucky in that regard, but she was kind of overprotective. She was apprehensive about me (her baby!) doing martial arts in the first place, so she was more than happy to see me quit. Besides, my parents didn't have much money and Tae Kwon Do was pretty expensive. It was win/win for her.

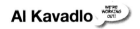

Al Kavadlo

Sometimes I wonder about how things might have been different if my mom had said to me what I am about to tell you. I suppose it probably wouldn't be all that different since I got into weight training soon after and had a new outlet with which I could explore the limits of my physical capabilities (and worry my mother). But, if it had been the Al of today sitting across from the twelve-year-old Al who wanted to quit Tae Kwon Do, I would have told him to toughen up! Anything that is worth doing is going to be hard at first. Everyone who is good at anything was bad at it at one point. We all have to start somewhere, no matter where that is. The only way to make progress is to keep doing it, even when it's hard. Even when you don't feel like it. Even when it sucks. I always have to remind my clients that our workouts aren't just about building muscle—they're about building character! Luckily, I still managed to learn this life lesson, in spite of weenie-ing out of Tae Kwon Do. So I guess you did all right, Mom.

A client of mine recently told me that she often feels anxious about what happens next in life. As she's saying this to me, she's doing lunges and getting sloppier with each rep. I remind her that if you focus on whatever you are doing right now, you'll be okay. You don't need to worry about the next moment; you'll be ready when it arrives. She smiled and got back to focusing on her workout. Her form improved and her anxiety melted away.

I believe we all have the power to shape our own destiny. It's just not as simple as some would want you to think. There is a key step in between thinking positively and getting what you want: TAKING ACTION! You can't just sit back and hope for good things, you have to go out there and work for them. I promise you this: if you seriously put in the time and effort (and don't kid yourself about it!), there is no way that you won't get results.

Instead of doubting your potential, embrace it. This isn't just about fitness; it's about your life. Take control of it and mold it into what you wish it to be. Remember, the only thing holding you back is you. Grab on to that feeling, the urge that made you read this book and ride it for all it's worth. Don't hesitate, act. Don't worry about the future, just concentrate on the now.

What are you waiting for? Put down the book because…WE'RE WORKING OUT!!!

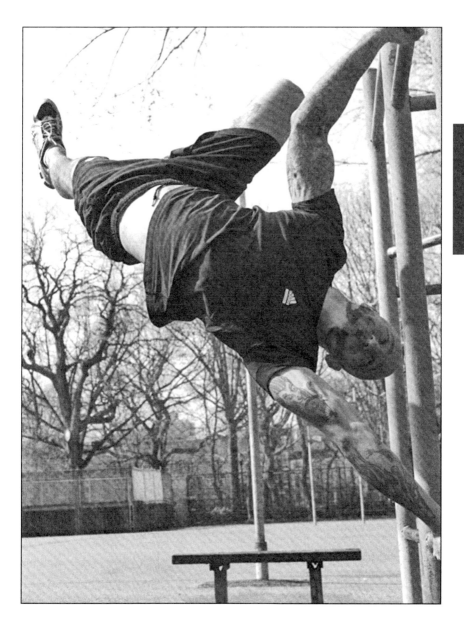

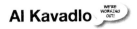

Appendix:
Sample Routines

What follows is a list of sample routines for full body strength training. For the no equipment routines and the jungle gym routines (which require a few bars of various heights and a bench or step), approach the sequence as a circuit, going through the exercises in order with as few breaks as possible. When you finish the circuit, take a breather (try to keep it under two minutes) then repeat the entire sequence. See how many times you can get through the routine in 30 minutes (without sacrificing proper form). As an alternative, you may approach these workouts from a traditional strength training perspective, doing each exercise for 2-4 consecutive sets with a short break in between each set (30-90 seconds). If you choose this method, the focus becomes more on strength and less on conditioning and endurance. They are both great approaches, but they will yield slightly different results. Experiment to find what works best for you and feel free to mix up the sequence of the exercises as you see fit. These are just guidelines, not strict prescriptions. I recommend that you watch the video clips on www.AlKavadlo.com for demonstrations and/or consult with a trainer to ensure safety.

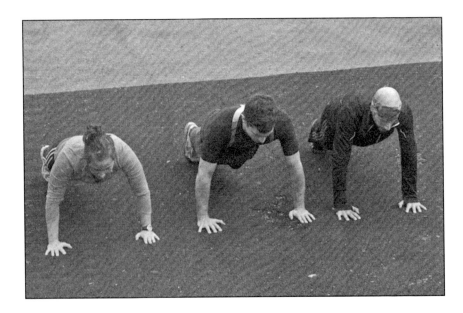

ROUTINES WITH NO EQUIPMENT

Beginner:
- Jumping jacks—20
- Squats—10
- Push-ups—10
- Stationary lunges—10 each leg
- Front plank—hold for 30 seconds
- Side plank—hold for 10 seconds each side

Intermediate:
- Jumping jacks—50
- Jump squats—10
- Plyo push-ups—10
- Stationary lunges—20 each leg
- Plank—hold for 60 seconds
- Side plank—hold for 30 seconds each side
- Handstand w/legs against wall—hold for 30 seconds

Advanced:
- Jumping jacks—100
- Pistol squats—10 each leg
- One arm push-ups —10 each arm
- Jumping lunges—10 each side
- Handstand—hold for 60 seconds
- Plank with one leg—hold for 60 seconds each leg
- Side plank with one leg—hold for 20 seconds each side

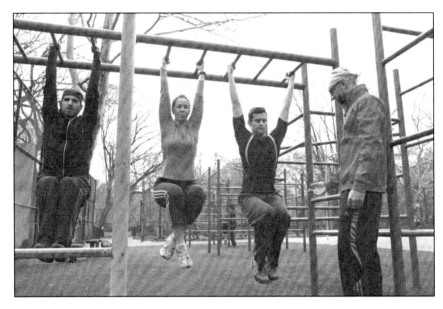

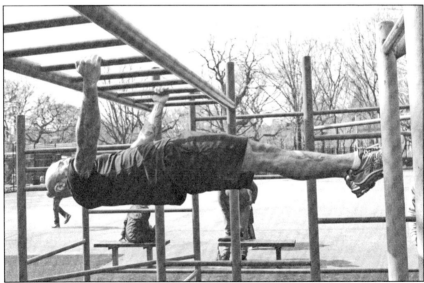

JUNGLE GYM WORKOUT—MINIMAL EQUIPMENT

Beginner:

- Hang from pull-up bar—hold for 30 seconds
- Push-ups—10
- Australian pull-ups—10
- Lunges—10 each leg
- Dips (on bench)—10
- Squats—10

Intermediate:

- Monkey bars—swing/climb across
- Plyo push-ups—10
- Pull-ups—8
- Step-ups onto bench—10 each leg
- Dips (on parallel bars)—10
- Walking lunges—20 each leg

Advanced:

- Muscle-ups—5
- Pistol squats—5 each leg
- Plyo push-ups—10
- Jumping lunges—5 each leg
- Plyo Australian pull-ups—10
- Jump-ups onto bench—10

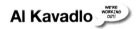

Al Kavadlo

GYM WORKOUT—BARBELLS, DUMBBELLS AND KETTLEBELLS

For the workouts below, perform each exercise for 2–4 sets of 6–10 repetitions each, with approximately one minute rest in between each set. If you want to add an additional cardio component you can perform active recovery between sets by doing jumping jacks, jumping rope or running in place. The amount of weight used will depend on your strength level. Challenge yourself by progressively building towards heavier weights over time, focusing primarily on keeping strict form. While I've labeled these routines Beginner, Intermediate and Advanced, they are all great workouts no matter how advanced you are (if you use enough weight!).

Beginner:
- Barbell squat
- Dumbbell or kettlebell lunge
- Barbell bench press
- Dumbbell or kettlebell bent-over row (on bench)
- Dumbbell or kettlebell overhead press
- Assisted pull-ups (or pull-down machine)

Intermediate:
- Barbell deadlift
- Kettlebell front squat
- Dumbbell step-up
- Dumbbell bench press
- Barbell overhead press
- Bent-over barbell row

Advanced:
- Barbell Romanian deadlift
- Barbell back lunge
- Barbell step-up

- Kettlebell windmill
- Weighted pull-ups
- Weighted dips

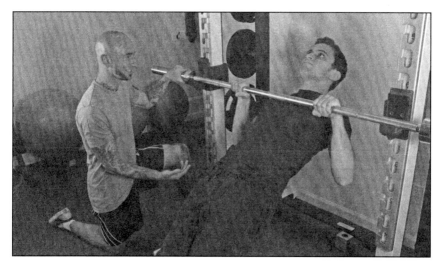

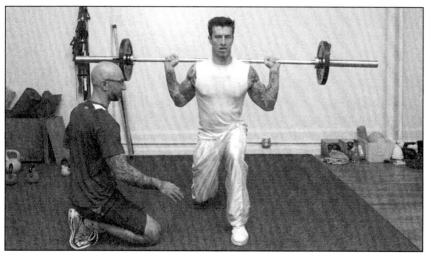

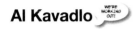
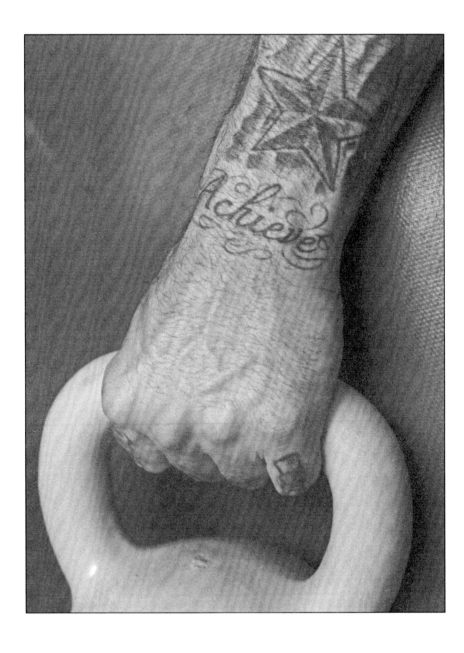